MW01003100

Landmark Cases in Forensic Psychiatry

Landmark Cases in Forensic Psychiatry

SECOND EDITION

Edited by

Merrill Rotter, MD

Director, Division of Law and Psychiatry
Associate Clinical Professor of Psychiatry
Albert Einstein School of Medicine
Bronx, New York

Jeremy Colley, MD

Associate Chief, Department of Psychiatry
Director, Division of Forensic Psychiatry
Bellevue Hospital Center
Associate Clinical Professor and
Program Director, Fellowship in Forensic Psychiatry
New York University School of Medicine

Heather Ellis Cucolo, ESQ

Owner, Mental Disability Law and Policy Associates
Adjunct Professor
New York Law School; Emory University School of Law

OXFORD
UNIVERSITY PRESS

Oxford University Press is a department of the University of Oxford. It furthers
the University's objective of excellence in research, scholarship, and education
by publishing worldwide. Oxford is a registered trade mark of Oxford University
Press in the UK and certain other countries.

Published in the United States of America by Oxford University Press
198 Madison Avenue, New York, NY 10016, United States of America.

© Oxford University Press 2019

First Edition published in 2014
Second Edition published in 2019

All rights reserved. No part of this publication may be reproduced, stored in
a retrieval system, or transmitted, in any form or by any means, without the
prior permission in writing of Oxford University Press, or as expressly permitted
by law, by license, or under terms agreed with the appropriate reproduction
rights organization. Inquiries concerning reproduction outside the scope of the
above should be sent to the Rights Department, Oxford University Press, at the
address above.

You must not circulate this work in any other form
and you must impose this same condition on any acquirer.

CIP data is on file at the Library of Congress
ISBN 978-0-19-091442-4

This material is not intended to be, and should not be considered, a substitute for medical or
other professional advice. Treatment for the conditions described in this material is highly
dependent on the individual circumstances. And, while this material is designed to offer
accurate information with respect to the subject matter covered and to be current as of the
time it was written, research and knowledge about medical and health issues is constantly
evolving and dose schedules for medications are being revised continually, with new side effects
recognized and accounted for regularly. Readers must therefore always check the product
information and clinical procedures with the most up-to-date published product information
and data sheets provided by the manufacturers and the most recent codes of conduct and safety
regulation. The publisher and the authors make no representations or warranties to readers,
express or implied, as to the accuracy or completeness of this material. Without limiting
the foregoing, the publisher and the authors make no representations or warranties as to
the accuracy or efficacy of the drug dosages mentioned in the material. The authors and the
publisher do not accept, and expressly disclaim, any responsibility for any liability, loss or risk
that may be claimed or incurred as a consequence of the use and/or application of any of the
contents of this material.

CONTENTS

ALPHABETICAL LIST OF CASES

CONTRIBUTORS

Eraka Bath, MD
Director, Child Forensic Services
Assistant Professor, Department of Psychiatry
UCLA Neuropsychiatric Institute
[Chapters 1, 11]

Jeremy Colley, MD
Associate Chief, Department of Psychiatry
Director, Division of Forensic Psychiatry
Bellevue Hospital Center
Associate Clinical Professor and
Program Director, Fellowship in Forensic Psychiatry
New York University School of Medicine
[Chapters 4, 21, 26, 27, 29, 30]

Heather Ellis Cucolo, ESQ
Owner, Mental Disability Law and Policy Associates
Adjunct Professor
New York Law School; Emory University School of Law
[Chapters 4, 16, 22, 23, 25, 26, 27, 29, 30]

Gregory Davis, MD
Attending Psychiatrist
Bellevue Hospital Center
Clinical Instructor in Psychiatry
New York University School of Medicine
[Chapter 2]

Elizabeth Ford, MD
Director, Division of Forensic Psychiatry
Bellevue Hospital Center
Training Director, Forensic Psychiatry Fellowship
Clinical Associate Professor of Psychiatry
New York University School of Medicine
[Chapters 6, 7, 13, 18]

Howard Forman, MD
Attending Physician
Division of Psychosomatic Medicine
Montefiore Medical Center
[Chapter 16]

Katya Frischer, MD
Associate Residency Director
Department of Psychiatry
Bronx Lebanon Hospital Center
Assistant Professor of Psychiatry
Albert Einstein College of Medicine of Yeshiva University
[Chapter 24]

Michael Greenspan, MD
Unit Chief
Zucker Hillside Hospital
North Shore–Long Island Jewish Health System
[Chapters 21, 23]

Matthew W. Grover, MD
Forensic Coordinator, Bronx Psychiatric Center
Associate Program Director, Forensic Psychiatry Fellowship
Assistant Clinical Professor of Psychiatry
Albert Einstein College of Medicine of Yeshiva University
[Chapter 22]

Omar Khan, MD
Attending Psychiatrist
Bellevue Hospital Center
Clinical Instructor in Psychiatry
New York University School of Medicine
[Chapter 25]

S. Shane Konrad, MD
Clinical Assistant Professor of Psychiatry
New York University School of Medicine
[Chapter 1]

Andrew M. Kopelman, MD
Attending Psychiatrist
Bellevue Hospital Center
Clinical Instructor in Psychiatry
New York University School of Medicine
[Chapter 3]

Li-Wen G. Lee, MD
Clinical Assistant Professor of Psychiatry
Columbia University College of Physicians and Surgeons
[Chapter 27]

Andrew P. Levin, MD
Assistant Clinical Professor of Psychiatry
Columbia University College of Physicians and Surgeons
[Chapter 19]

Rebecca Lewis, MD
Clinical Instructor in Psychiatry
New York University School of Medicine
[Chapters 9, 25]

Amar Mehta, MD
Forensic Psychiatrist
San Quentin State Prison
[Chapters 17, 21]

Merrill Rotter, MD
Director, Division of Law and Psychiatry
Associate Clinical Professor of Psychiatry
Albert Einstein College of Medicine
[Chapters 16, 18, 19, 20, 21, 22, 23, 26, 27, 30]

Eileen P. Ryan, DO
Associate Professor of Psychiatry and Neurobehavioral Sciences
University of Virginia School of Medicine
[Chapters 12, 13]

Bryan C. Shelby, MD, JD
Attending Psychiatrist, Substance Abuse Treatment Program
Newington Veterans Hospital
Assistant Professor of Psychiatry
University of Connecticut Health Center School of Medicine
[Chapters 4, 18]

Shawn S. Sidhu, MD
Inpatient Attending Psychiatrist, Children's
    Psychiatric Center
Assistant Professor, University of New Mexico Department
    of Psychiatry
[Chapters 11, 14]

Scott Soloway, MD
Director, Manhattan/Correctional Assisted Outpatient
    Treatment Program
New York City Department of Health and Mental Hygiene
Clinical Assistant Professor of Psychiatry
New York University School of Medicine
[Chapter 4]

Tara Straka, MD
Attending Psychiatrist, Kirby Forensic Psychiatric Center
Clinical Instructor in Psychiatry
New York University School of Medicine
[Chapter 26]

Bipin Subedi, MD
Clinical Instructor in Psychiatry
New York University School of Medicine
[Chapters 8, 25]

INTRODUCTION

MERRILL ROTTER, JEREMY COLLEY, HEATHER ELLIS CUCOLO, AND ELIZABETH FORD

Forensic psychiatry (the interface of psychiatry and the law), forensic psychology, and mental health law are growing and evolving subspecialties in their respective larger disciplines. The fields are deeply rooted in the written opinions and holdings about mental health from various U.S. courts (with one exception—*M'Naghten's Case* of 1843), most important, the U.S. Supreme Court. These decisions cover topics as broad-reaching as informed consent and as narrow as sentencing guidelines for adolescents convicted of nonhomicide cases. The opinions are frequently lengthy and dense, with much revealed in the writing not only about the specific reasoning behind a decision but also about the sociopolitical climate at the time of the case and the political preferences of the appointed justices on the bench. The opinions can read easily like novels or more laboriously like legal textbooks. Regardless of the style or length, however, the substance of the decision is critical for some facet of the mental health system in this country. Without knowledge of the historical and legal precedents set by these cases, mental health practitioners are at a significant disadvantage.

Recognizing the importance of these holdings, the American Academy of Psychiatry and the Law (AAPL), the premier national organization in the United States for forensic psychiatrists, compiled a list of more than 100 cases representing the core of the specialty. Because the list was created more than 25 years ago, it has changed as new cases have been decided and others have become obsolete or outdated. The last update was published in 2014.[1] However, the majority of the decisions remain essential to understanding why practitioners in mental health are legally required to practice as they do. Most, if not all, of the 45 American and 8 Canadian forensic psychiatry fellowship training programs, competitive subspecialty training programs available after completion of a 4-year psychiatry residency, incorporate discussion and study of the landmark cases into their year-long didactics.

The American Board of Forensic Psychiatry was founded in 1976 to establish standards for competence in psychiatry and the law. The board administered its own examination and certified 253 diplomates until the American Board of Medical Specialties officially recognized the field of forensic psychiatry in 1992.[2] Since then, the American Board of Psychiatry and Neurology (ABPN) has been certifying specialists in the field of forensic psychiatry (the ABPN administered its first exam in 1994) and continues to sponsor a biannual written certification exam. Passing this increasingly rigorous exam following completion of a forensic psychiatry fellowship is considered evidence of one's competence and professionalism in the field and, much like general board certification in other areas of medicine, is a highly coveted accomplishment. Recertification is required every 10 years to maintain standing with the ABPN. The American Board of Forensic Psychology also administers a certification exam for forensic psychologists and has done so since 1947. Unlike the ABPN, this certification also involves work review and an oral examination.[3]

The emphasis that the ABPN certification and recertification exams have placed on knowledge of the landmark cases has evolved over the years. While various exams have encouraged or discouraged rote memorization of case names and jurisdictions, the impact of the holdings and accompanying reasoning on the practice of forensic psychiatry has always remained critical. In January 2013, the ABPN published a Content Outline for its 200-question, multiple-choice certification examination and highlighted the key areas of knowledge required. Included in that outline are 100 landmark cases covering the legal regulation of psychiatry, civil and criminal issues, the death penalty, corrections and correctional health care, basic law, children and family issues, and special issues in forensic psychiatry.[4]

Sources of study for landmark cases have typically taken the form of a compilation of summaries and/or discussion of cases in forensic psychiatry textbooks,[5,6] in mental health law texts,[6,7,8] and in the course materials for the annual 3-day American Academy of Psychiatry and the Law Forensic Psychiatry Review Course.[9] A set of landmark case "flash cards" was available for a brief period (2005–2010) that had been created by the New York University Forensic Psychiatry Fellowship Class of 2005.[10] The majority of the texts of the opinions themselves are easily accessible online. While this collection of sources is and will continue to be extremely useful, and was invaluable in the preparation of this book, it does not uniquely focus on the landmark cases (with the exception of the defunct flash cards and the lengthy court opinions) in a way that is clearly aimed at both developing a greater understanding of their impact and preparing for an examination. This book was written to fill that gap.

We have designed this book with forensic psychiatry and psychology trainees and practicing clinicians in mind. There are six sections that define broad topic areas, included in which are multiple chapters with more narrow areas of focus. We classified cases based on our interpretation of the most important holding for each case. While this classification system tends to align with the way other sources have grouped cases, there are some changes that we think will help the reader better contextualize the narrative and practical implications of the cases. The AAPL grouping can be accessed online.[1]

All the cases listed in the 2015 ABPN Content Outline are included, as are other cases that we find particularly important for understanding a topic. Not all the cases will seem relevant, and indeed some have been overturned by higher rulings, but when preparing for a board exam, we find it better to be more inclusive rather than less.

We have tried to create summaries that are easy to follow and get quickly to the point. They are presented chronologically in each chapter so that the reader can understand the evolution of ideas on a particular topic. We have also turned the main holding of each case into a "yes or no" question to allow readers to get even more quickly to the point. Bear in mind that in order to provide concise summaries for study purposes, many of the details of each individual case have been excluded. For those who would like to review the cases in more detail, we have provided a free online link to the full text of each case.

Although this study guide is not designed in any way to be a primer on law or the legal system, the cases discussed have all been adjudicated within the context of state or federal court systems, most frequently the U.S. Supreme Court. This body is the highest federal court in the United States and has as a major task deciding cases for which it grants certiorari (a willingness to hear a case) based on an interpretation of the U.S. Constitution. The Bill of Rights (the first 10 amendments to the Constitution, ratified in 1791) and the Fourteenth Amendment form the basis for Court's decisions involving psychiatry and are listed in Appendix A. Appendices B and C present a very general framework about state and federal court systems in the United States. It is not necessary to know the exact path a case took to get to the Supreme Court, but the various arguments presented along the way for and against a particular outcome are important. It is also useful to know to which jurisdiction a case applies (e.g., only a particular state district, all of the states represented in a court of appeals circuit). In this edition, we have added a glossary of words, terms, and phrases commonly found in landmark cases (Appendix D).

The addition of a robust assembly of multiple-choice questions at the end of each section will help test the reader's knowledge and test-taking skills; we hope the detailed explanations of each answer will also help cement that knowledge in a lasting way. The questions are designed to mimic ABPN-style questions (e.g., no "except" questions, no "A and B, A and C" answers) but should be used only for guidance and practice. The questions are not drawn from actual board exams but have been created by the editors and contributors to be as clear and as helpful as possible.

While the AAPL Landmark Case list has not been updated since 2014 and the most recent ABPN content outline (published 2015) does not include any new landmark cases, we have created this second edition with two primary goals in mind: (1) to ensure that the landmark case summaries contain the most accurate and up-to-date information; the cases may not change, but their relevance may have, and (2) to include additional cases, which never did or may not yet have obtained landmark case status, but we believe are relevant to current practice of forensic psychiatry; these include some new cases in existing sections, as well as new chapters on immigration and gun ownership. The additional cases which have not been accorded landmark status (according to AAPL and the ABPN) at the time of this publication are indicated in the table of contents. The only cases that were eliminated in this second edition are those dealing with ERISA, the federal regulations regarding health insurance that are no longer particularly influential or relevant.

Finally, as noted earlier, within each chapter, the cases are presented in chronological order so as to enhance the clarity of law's evolution. In this edition, we have included a new conceptual chapter, The Forensic Psychiatry Paper Chase: The Case for the Landmark Case Seminar. In this chapter, the authors provide further evidence for how, when seen from a chronological perspective, the study of landmark cases can demonstrate how the cases influence one another and illuminate the social, political, and legal developments that have influenced the practice of forensic psychiatry.

The editors of the second edition are grateful to all of the authors who contributed to the original book. Also a special thank you to Dr. Elizabeth Ford, who coedited the first edition and who continues to provide creative and inspirational leadership in teaching and practicing forensic psychiatry.

REFERENCES

1. *Landmark Cases 2014*. Retrieved from http://aapl.org/landmark-cases.
2. Prentice, S. E. (1995). A history of subspecialization in forensic psychiatry. *Bulletin of the American Academy of Psychiatry Law*, 23(2), 195–203.
3. American Board of Forensic Psychology. http://www.abfp.com/brochure.asp. Accessed November 6, 2013.

4. ABPN. Subspecialty Certification Examination in Forensic Psychiatry, 2013 Content Blueprint. www.abpn.com/downloads/content_outlines/Initial Cert/ 2013-FP-blueprint-010413-EE-MR.pdf. Issued January 4, 2013.
5. Rosner, R, ed. (2003). *Principles and practice of forensic psychiatry* (2nd ed.). London: Arnold.
6. Simon, R. I., & Gold, L. (2010). *Textbook of forensic psychiatry* (2nd ed.). Arlington, VA: American Psychiatric Publishing.
7. Perlin, M. I. (2005). *Mental disability law: Cases and materials* (2nd ed.). Durham, NC: Carolina Academic Press.
8. Slobogin, C., & Rai, A. (2008). *Law and the mental health system: Civil and criminal aspects* (5th ed.). St. Paul, MN: West Academic Publishing.
9. Resnick, P. (2012). *Annual forensic psychiatry review course.* Bloomfield, CT: American Academy of Psychiatry and the Law.
10. Ford, E., Bath, E., Lopez-Leon, M., & Soloway, S. (2008). *Flash Forensics TM: U.S. landmark cases about psychiatry and the law* (2nd ed.). New York.

The Forensic Psychiatry Paper Chase

Making the Case for the Landmark Cases Seminar

MERRILL ROTTER, JEREMY COLLEY,
HEATHER ELLIS CUCOLO, ELIZABETH FORD,
AND HOWARD FORMAN

Every few years the American Academy of Psychiatry and the Law (AAPL) reviews and "selects Landmark Cases which it thinks are especially important and significant for forensic psychiatry."[1] For training purposes, "significant for forensic society" may mean that the case retains continuing legal relevance or has significant historical importance. Pedagogically, these cases can be taught to forensic psychiatrists as part of content-specific seminars that reference the relevant holding, as in a lecture on civil commitment that notes the changes brought via the case of *O'Connor v. Donaldson*,[2] or a review of legal insanity that references the M'Naghten standard. Alternatively, the cases can be taught as a stand-alone seminar. In this chapter, we review the advantages of this latter approach.

The Accreditation Council for Graduate Medical Education (ACGME) requirements for Graduate Medical Education in Forensic Psychiatry include demonstrating competence in "ethical, administrative, and legal issues in forensic psychiatry...history of forensic psychiatry...roles and responsibilities of forensic psychiatrists . . . basic civil procedure . . . basic criminal procedure . . . fundamentals of law, statutes, and administrative regulations . . . jurisdiction...fundamentals of law, statutes, and administrative regulations."[3] While none of these require a separate curriculum in Landmark Cases, we will argue herein that all of these—as well as the many, if not all, of the other required substantive content areas—can be significantly enhanced by an approach that places said content in its original legal context. There is an imperfect fit between what the law requires and what forensic psychiatry seeks to achieve. The law requires an ultimate conclusion—a black-and-white, dyadic final assessment—while psychiatry rarely deals in finalities and is an ever-growing and changing field. Oftentimes, certain areas of the law require input from the clinical community and statutory language can require psychiatrists to assist the fact finder (judge or jury) in making the ultimate decision in the fate of an individual. Psychiatrists who choose to step into the legal arena would greatly benefit by studying the specific facts of a case and the legal rationale associated with a particular holding to illuminate the historical, social, clinical, ethical, and legal considerations in a way that is not possible through a mere limited review.

Through a Landmark Case seminar, students explore legal opinions which reflect the evolution and roots of forensic psychiatry throughout its historical development, as well as the relationship between psychiatry and broad social and legal trends, including civil rights, federalism, law enforcement, and the role of government in serving or supporting underserved populations with and without mental illness. In addition, these legal opinions, which we rely on as clinicians and forensic psychiatrists, are often themselves based on the understanding (or misunderstanding) of the state of the art/science at the time of the decision, for example, the relevance and appropriate use of psychoanalytic principles, the risks and benefits of psychopharmacologic treatment, the reliability of dangerousness predictions, and the clinical utility of milieu therapy.[4]

In particular, a chronologic review of landmark cases allows these trends to emerge naturally, while also demonstrating the importance of precedence and critical legal concepts.[5] In this chapter we demonstrate these important goals by outlining the cases and principles that would be traced through the landmark case list. To further illustrate the utility of the in-depth, case-based approach, we review *Jackson v. Indiana*[6] and *Addington v. Texas*,[7] and we identify examples of how a case can evolve from its origin as a landmark case to one that is later cited to highlight an important legal principle, although not necessarily the specific holding of the original case. Finally, judicial clarifications of the concept of liberty and judicial perspectives on clinical psychiatry provide examples of how legal and clinical trends naturally emerge and are reinforced through a standalone, chronological review of complete landmark case opinions.

METHODS

Senior forensic psychiatrists with experience in writing and teaching landmark case–related material reviewed the 130 cases listed by the AAPL as of

2014.[1] Each reviewer was asked to identify any prior landmark cases cited by the majority opinion and the specific legal issue for which it was cited. The number of times each landmark case was cited was tallied, as were the number of references to specific legal issues. A consensus decision making was utilized to identify the common legal issues in the cases to maximize consistency and reliability.

RESULTS

Tables 1.1 and 1.2 list, respectively, the landmark cases and the legal principles that were cited at least five times. The demonstrated repetition of cases and principles provides for the pedagogic opportunity described earlier. Reviewing landmark cases in chronological order allows students to witness the importance of precedence, see firsthand how earlier cases are mined for similarities and differences in fact pattern and legal principle, identify the sometimes surprising ways in which a case may be used in a court's reasoning, while simultaneously reinforcing details and holdings of some of the most important cases; *Jackson*[6] and *Addington*[7] will be described as examples of this type of analysis. (See Tables 1.3 and 1.4, respectively.) In an analogous fashion, one can trace a legal principle through the various cases in which it is referenced and, importantly, the various meanings it may take on in each new case. (See Table 1.5.)

JACKSON V. INDIANA (1972)

In *Jackson v. Indiana*,[6] Theon Jackson was a mentally retarded, deaf, mute individual, incapable of reading, writing, or communicating in any way

Table 1.1 LANDMARK CASE (NO. OF SUBSEQUENT CITATIONS)

Robinson v. California (11)
O'Connor v. Donaldson (11)
Addington v. Texas (11)
Jackson v. Indiana (10)
Vitek v. Jones (10)
Youngberg v. Romeo (10)
Baxstrom v. Herold (6)
Tarasoff v. Regents of U. of Cal. (5)
Sup. of Belchertown v. Saikowitz (5)

Table 1.2 LEGAL PRINCIPLE (NO. OF REFERENCES)
Liberty (37)
Evolving standards of the Eighth Amendment (17)
State interests vs. individual rights (18)
What constitutes procedural due process (13)
Uncertainty about psychiatry (16)
Confinement related to purpose (8)
State interest in safety (5)
Definition of case as civil vs. criminal (5)
Equal protection (5)

except through a limited knowledge of sign language, who was indicted on two counts of robbery (apparently both involving purse snatches). Notwithstanding testimony at his competency hearing that it was doubtful that Jackson could ever learn to read or write or become proficient in sign language, and that it would be impossible for him to learn minimal communications skills in an Indiana state institution, Jackson was committed indefinitely to a state *hospital* "until such time as [the state] should certify to the court that the '*defendant is sane*'" (*Jackson* at 719, emphasis added). Jackson brought suit challenging his confinement under the original criminal law competency-based standards, citing violation of the Eighth Amendment prohibition against cruel and unusual punishment, as well as the Fourteenth Amendment guarantees of due process and equal protection. The U.S. Supreme Court held that inasmuch as Mr. Jackson was not likely to be restored to competence to stand trial, the purpose for his initial confinement was no longer valid and the mere fact of his arrest was not a legally relevant distinguishing feature between him and others subject to involuntary hospitalization. The U.S. Supreme Court found that both the Due Process Clause governed all matters related to the "nature and duration" of a commitment term. Therefore, his continued confinement would have to meet the legal requirements for civil commitment, including a finding of dangerousness to self or others, which was not part of the criminal incompetency standard.

Among subsequent landmark cases addressing competency to stand trial, *Cooper v. Oklahoma*[8] most specifically references the *Jackson*, holding that there should be a reasonable restriction on the length of time a person can be held to be made or found competent, although that reference was not critical to its actual holding. In making it easier for an

Table 1.3 *JACKSON V. INDIANA* (1972)

Year	Case	Reference
1975	*O'Connor v. Donaldson*	The fact that state law may have authorized confinement of the harmless mentally ill does not itself establish a constitutionally adequate purpose for the confinement. ... even if his involuntary confinement was initially permissible, it could not constitutionally continue after that basis no longer existed.
1977	*Fasulo v. Arafeh*	Commitment must be justified on the basis of a legitimate state interest.... Equally important confinement must cease when those reasons no longer exist.
1979	*Addingtion v. Texas*	This Court repeatedly has recognized that civil commitment for any purpose constitutes a significant deprivation of liberty that requires due process protection.
1980	*Vitek v. Jones*	Our cases recognize as much, and reflect an understanding that involuntary commitment to a mental hospital is not within the range of conditions of confinement to which a prison sentence subjects an individual.
1990	*Cruzan v. Dir. Missouri DMH*	Nor does the fact that Nancy Cruzan is now incompetent deprive her of her fundamental rights.
1993	*Godinez v. Moran*	Competency for one purpose does not necessarily translate to competency for another purpose.
1997	*Kansas v. Hendricks*	... the Court itself has used a variety of expressions to describe the mental condition of those properly subject to civil confinement.

individual to be found incompetent, the Court noted that any concerns about malingering (i.e., an erroneous finding of incompetence) could be uncovered and remedied in the course of the subsequent restoration-focused treatment.

More on point in applying *Jackson,* in *Godinez v. Moran,*[9] the dissent wanted to distinguish between various competencies (e.g., stand trial, plead guilty, represent self). The dissenting Justices quoted Jackson, and, in turn *Jackson*'s own citation of *Drope v. Missouri*[10] that "a defendant's mental condition may be relevant to more than one legal issue, each governed by distinct rules reflecting quite different policies."

Table 1.4 ADDINGTON V. TEXAS (1972)

Year	Case	Reference
1980	*Vitek v. Jones*	It is indisputable that commitment to a mental hospital "can engender adverse social consequences to the individual" and that "whether we label this phenomena 'stigma' or choose to call it something else . . . we recognize that it can occur and that it can have a very significant impact on the individual."
1982	*Youngberg v. Romeo*	In that case, we held that the State must prove the need for commitment by "clear and convincing" evidence. We reached this decision by weighing the individual's liberty interest against the State's legitimate interests in confinement.
1983	*Barefoot v. Estelle*	There may be factual issues in a commitment proceeding, but the factual aspects represent only the beginning of the inquiry. Whether the individual is mentally ill and dangerous to either himself or others and is in need of confined therapy turns on the meaning of the facts which must be interpreted by expert psychiatrists and psychologists.
1983	*Rennie v. Klein*	The individual should not be asked to share equally with society the risk of error when the possible injury to the individual is significantly greater than any possible harm to the state.
1983	*JR v. Parham*	In terms of public reaction, the child who exhibits abnormal behavior may be seriously injured by an erroneous decision not to commit. Appellees overlook a significant source of the public reaction to the mentally ill, for what is truly "stigmatizing" is the symptomatology of a mental or emotional illness.
1984	*In re: Richardson*	[O]ne who is suffering from a debilitating mental illness and in need of treatment is neither wholly at liberty nor free of stigma.
1986	*Allen v. Illinois*	Civil commitment state power is not exercised in a punitive sense.
1986	*Ford v. Wainwright*	And unlike the determination of whether the death penalty is appropriate in a particular case, the competency determination depends substantially on expert analysis in a discipline fraught with "subtleties and nuances."
1989	*Cruzan v. Director*	The function of a standard of proof, as that concept is embodied in the Due Process Clause and in the realm of factfinding, is to "instruct the factfinder concerning the degree of confidence our society thinks he should have in the correctness of factual conclusions for a particular type of adjudication."

Table 1.4 CONTINUED

Year	Case	Reference
1990	*Zinermon v. Burch*	Civil commitment for any purpose constitutes a significant deprivation of liberty that requires due process protection.
1992	*Riggins v. Nevada*	The Due Process Clause allows civil commitment of individuals shown by clear and convincing evidence to be mentally ill and dangerous.
1993	U.S. *v. Jones*	Proof that the acquittee committed a criminal act as a result of mental illness eliminates the risk that he is being committed for mere idiosyncratic behavior.
1997	*Kansas v. Hendricks*	The psychiatric debate, therefore, helps to inform the law by setting the bounds of what is reasonable, but it cannot here decide just how States must write their laws within those bounds.
2002	*Kansas v. Crane*	Nor, when considering civil commitment, have we ordinarily distinguished for constitutional purposes among volitional, emotional, and cognitive impairments.

In addition, however, there are references to *Jackson* in cases that go beyond issues related to competency to stand trial. *Jackson* is yet another case cited by the majority and/or dissent in establishing that involuntary hospitalization is a severe deprivation of liberty.[2,7,11,12] However, *Jackson* is also cited to support the concept that in specific contexts a legitimate state interest may override this liberty interest.[13,14] And yet, in *O'Connor v. Donaldson*,[2] the U.S. Supreme Court is more tempered.

Jackson is again referenced as part of a justification for the Court's review of Florida civil commitment law as applied to Mr. Donaldson as part of the legal justification for the idea that despite the principle of deferring to legitimate state interests, the constitutional guarantee of liberty may call into question and trump traditional state sovereignty and statutes governing involuntary confinement.

Jackson also provides a precedent for the idea that while liberty may be restricted by confinement on criminal grounds, clinically driven civil commitment is a distinguishable loss, requiring additional or different due process.[15] Whether the confinement is deemed civil or criminal, *Jackson*'s most all-encompassing principle regarding the appropriate balance between individual liberty and state interest is one quoted in several subsequent landmark cases: "at the very least, due process requires that the nature and duration of commitment bear some reasonable relation to the purpose for which the individual is committed."[6]

Table 1.5

Definitions of Liberty	Uncertainty Regarding Psychiatry
Freedom from	Psychiatric Diagnosis
Physical confinement	Predictions of Dangerousness
Physical restraint	
Stigma	• Capital punishment
Unsafe conditions of state confinement	• Civil commitment of adults
Unsafe conditions due to state policies	• Civil commitment of minors
Unwanted treatment	• Treatment decisions for inpatients
Mental illness	
Freedom of choice	

Finally, *Jackson* is referenced in cases far from the rights of an incompetent, deaf, mute defendant with intellectual deficiency, including cases involving issues of the right to die and sex offender commitment. As part of its opinion in the right-to-die case of *Cruzan v. Director, Missouri DMH*,[16] the Court cites *Jackson* and notes that liberty interests survive even when the individual in question has already been found incompetent. The sex offender civil commitment case *Kansas v. Hendricks*[17] reached back to *Jackson* in finding that a legislature had the power to define the term "mental abnormality." The majority noted that psychiatrists often disagree about how to define "mental illness." The Court goes on to assert that there are "a variety of expressions to describe [a] mental condition," and *Jackson* is one among a number of cases in which the Court has recognized other terms for mental illness, including "incompetency" and "insanity."

ADDINGTON V. TEXAS (1979)

Mr. Frank O'Neal Addington[7] challenged his civil commitment, arguing that the standard of proof in Texas at the time—clear and convincing evidence of dangerousness secondary to mental illness—violated the Fourteenth Amendment by not affording adequate due process; Addington argued that the criminal standard of proof—beyond a reasonable doubt—should apply. The case wound its way through the Texas courts, with the state supreme court opining that instead of beyond a reasonable doubt or clear and convincing, the appropriate standard ought to be preponderance of the evidence. Both the state and Addington appealed, and the U.S. Supreme Court granted certiorari.

The Court acknowledged that avoiding civil commitment represents a substantial liberty interest, and that one of the fundamental principles guiding determinations of standard of proof is managing the risk of erroneous decisions. The stakes surrounding involuntary commitment are graver than seeking monetary damages via torts, and, therefore, the Court argued that mere preponderance of the evidence is not an appropriate standard. On the other hand, involuntary commitment, at least in part, is for the purposes of treatment, not punishment, and, therefore, the standard of proof of beyond a reasonable doubt is too stringent. In addition, the Court commented on the uncertainty of psychiatric diagnosis and predictions of dangerousness, saying that psychiatrists would never be able to provide opinions with such confidence as to reach the standard of beyond a reasonable doubt. Therefore, the Court decided that clear and convincing provides adequate due process protections.

Not surprisingly, *Addington* is cited liberally in cases regarding due process protections involving civil commitment in various contexts, such as *Zinermon v. Burch* (due process for "voluntary" civil commitment),[11] *Vitek v. Jones* (transport of felons from prison to a psychiatric facility),[15] *Kansas v. Hendricks*,[17] *Jones v. U.S.* (commitment of insanity acquitees),[18] *Riggins v. Nevada* (commitment for incompetence to stand trial),[19] *Allen v. Illinois*,[20] and *Kansas v. Crane* (civil commitment of sexually violent predators).[21] It is also frequently cited in cases involving other deprivations of liberty involving the mentally ill, as in *Youngberg v. Romeo* (freedom from restraint)[22] and *Rennie v. Klein* (freedom from forced medication).[23]

However, *Addington* is also cited in subsequent cases for some of its subtler points and reasoning, with regards to how the courts mitigate against erroneous decisions, in general, and, more specifically, with regards to the notion of stigma as it relates to mental illness. In *Addington*, the Court argued for the need for robust due process protections to protect citizens from being civilly committed for mere "idiosyncratic behavior," observing that being labeled falsely as mentally ill represented a deprivation of liberty beyond simply being confined. In *Parham v. JR*,[24] the Court cites *Addington*, but elaborates that stigma can also manifest if a person who is mentally ill is *not* committed, as the person, though not confined, will continue to show signs and symptoms of his illness to the public. This theme continues: In *re: Richardson*,[25] in quoting *Addington*: "[o]ne who is suffering from a debilitating mental illness and in need of treatment is neither wholly at liberty nor free of stigma."

In an interesting twist, *Ford v. Wainwright*[26] uses *Addington* in its argument against the right to a judicial determination of sanity to undergo execution, as it selectively quotes *Addington*'s characterization of psychiatry as "a discipline fraught with 'subtleties and nuances.'" *Addington* makes this comment in the context of arguing that the standard of proof of beyond a reasonable doubt is too high for civil commitment, but *Ford* pivots the concept through *Parham*, which, as described earlier, to opine that children facing civil commitment do not have a right to judicial review, a debate that was not at issue in *Addington* itself.

Cruzan[16] adopts *Addington*'s reasoning process to support its determination that the State of Missouri could require the parents of Nancy Cruzan to prove by clear and convincing evidence that their daughter, if competent, would have requested cessation of nutrition and hydration. *Addington* said that a standard of proof of clear and convincing informed the finder of fact of the relative importance of the deprivation of liberty, in the face of the state's interest. Though *Addington* was not about medical decision making or end-of-life care, the principles it outlined regarding balancing individual liberties with regards to diagnosis of mental illness and commitment translated well to questions in front of the *Cruzan* court.

LIBERTY

. . . nor shall any state deprive any person of life, liberty, or property, without due process of law
—Fourteenth Amendment[27]

First cited as an aspiration in the Declaration of Independence,[28] along with life and the pursuit of happiness, liberty came to be most explicitly and relevantly codified as a legal principle in the Fourteenth Amendment of the Constitution wherein the State is precluded from depriving "any person of life, liberty of property without due process of law." In an 1897 insurance case, the U.S. Supreme Court declared that liberty "means not only the right of the citizen to be free from the mere physical restraint of his person, as by incarceration, but the term is deemed to embrace the right of the citizen to be free in the enjoyment of all his faculties, to be free to use them in all lawful ways, to live and work where he will . . . "[29]

In our landmark case review, it is, by far, the most frequently referenced legal principle. As one traces the concept of liberty through the cases, it takes on very varied, and occasionally surprisingly expansive meanings. When broadly conceptualized as freedom—freedom of movement, freedom of choice, freedom from unwanted medical intrusion, freedom from the limiting effects of being stigmatized, freedom to exercise autonomy—these meanings are not as surprising as they may initially appear.

. . . to confine a person for compulsory psychiatric treatment [is] massive curtailment of liberty . . . [30]

All civil commitment cases most obviously impact an individual's liberty interest inasmuch as they allow for a person to be held against his will. Not surprisingly therefore, cases delineating the necessary substantive due process criteria such as *O'Connor v. Donaldson* ("ability to survive safely in the community"),[2] and procedural criteria such as *Addington v. Texas* ("clear and convincing evidence" standard)[7] call for this high-level specificity and confidence to achieve the proper respect for and protection of the liberty interest of an individual subject to civil commitment.

The loss of liberty produced by an involuntary commitment is more than a loss of freedom from confinement.[15]

Less obviously, civil commitment may be an even more concerning loss of liberty than correctional incarceration. The liberty interest in avoiding un-wanted stigma and avoiding involuntary treatment associated with civil commitment exists even for an inmate whose freedoms—particularly freedom of movement and choice—have already been restricted by the crim-inal conviction and sentence. In *Vitek v. Jones*[15] and *Baxstrom v. Herold*,[31] cur-rent or recent incarceration provided no exception to the need for a hearing on involuntary hospitalization. In *Washington v. Harper*,[12] despite being a sentenced prisoner, Harper was found to require some (though not court-based) due process, given his continuing liberty interest in avoiding the ad-ditional intrusion of unwanted medication. In fact, the quote cited earlier describing civil commitment as a "massive curtailment of liberty" comes, not from a civil law case, but rather from *Humphrey v. Cady*,[30] another case involving an individual subject to confinement under criminal law.

To go from a state of confinement to confinement plus forced medication involves a major change in the conditions of confinement[15]

Liberty interests clearly survive even the "massive curtailment" associated with involuntary hospitalization. In *Youngberg v. Romeo*,[22] *Clites v. Iowa*,[32] and *Jackson v. Indiana*,[6] the U.S. Supreme Court noted that even a person already subject to civil commitment has a liberty interest in being free from restraints, a further limitation on physical movement. In *Youngberg*, the freedom to live in a safe environment was also characterized as a liberty in-terest (although in a later case, *Deshaney v. Winnebago County Dept. of Social Services*,[33] the majority opinion of the Court suggested that in *Youngberg*, the state's duty to provide safety stemmed from the initial deprivation of liberty by the state, i.e., the involuntary hospitalization). And despite the involuntariness of their hospitalization, civilly committed persons retain a liberty interest in freedom from being given medication involuntarily, because of the physical intrusion it presents, as well as because of the intrusion on the autonomy to make the choice not to take medication.[13,23,34]

The limitations on the liberty to make autonomous choices and to act on those choices when deprived of liberty (e.g., hospitalization or incarceration) is cited as the justification for the state's having, at least, some minimal constitutional duty to provide care and safety.[22,35] In *Deshaney*, a child abuse case, the argument about liberty between the majority and dissent turns, in part, on whether the state, in establishing a system for child abuse reporting and remediation, had effectively "confined" the abused child in the care of the father, and thus taken on a duty to protect him.[33]

To presume that the incompetent person must always be subjected to what many rational and intelligent persons may decline is to downgrade the status of the incompetent person by placing a lesser value on his intrinsic human worth and vitality.[36]

It is not surprising that liberty interests survive even when there has been loss of liberty associated with incarceration and hospitalization. Courts have been clear even when a person is presumptively incompetent they retain liberty interest that must be taken into consideration. This includes children,[24] adults who came to be in persistent vegetative states,[16] and even those who never had an opportunity to exercise any autonomy due to profound development disability.[36]

That many of the rights and liberties protected by the Due Process Clause sound in personal autonomy does not warrant the sweeping conclusion that any and all important, intimate, and personal decisions are so protected.[37]

Liberty defined as the exercise of autonomous choice was at the heart of non–civil commitment cases, including *Washington v. Glucksburg*[37] and *Vacco v. Quill*,[38] in which the Court affirmed the idea that protection of liberty includes an individual's right to autonomous decision making, but further clarified that the type of choice (assisted suicide in these two cases) was part of defining whether the specific choice was a constitutionally guaranteed liberty interest; assisted suicide was deemed not to be such a choice.

One who is suffering from a debilitating mental illness and in need of treatment is neither wholly at liberty nor free of stigma.[7]

Finally, as the Supreme Court observed in *Addington v. Texas*,[7] a person with mental illness may not be entirely free, even if spared the intrusive limitation of civil commitment, because mental illness itself, with its associated assault on autonomous decision making, represents a loss of liberty. The majority cited a 1976 article by Chodoff, in which he wrote, " . . . is freedom defined only by the absence of external restraints? Internal physiological or psychological processes can contribute to the throttling of the spirit that is as painful as any applied from the outside,"[39] they could equally convincingly have reached back to 1897 and cited themselves in *Allgeyer v. Louisiana*: if liberty, as defined in that case, is the freedom to "the enjoyment one's faculties," then is one truly at liberty if those very faculties are constrained by symptoms of mental illness?[29]

UNCERTAINTY ABOUT PSYCHIATRY

When is it, one must wonder, that the psychotherapist came to play such an indispensable role in the maintenance of the citizenry's mental health? For most of history, men and women have worked out their difficulties by talking to, inter alios, parents, siblings, best friends, and bartenders. . . Ask the average citizen: Would your mental health be more significantly impaired by preventing you from seeing a psychotherapist, or by preventing you from getting advice from your mom?[40]

The courts, while consistently acknowledging psychiatry as a legitimate branch of medicine, and relying on the expertise of psychiatrists to help the finder of fact, have just as consistently articulated skepticism of the field, as echoed in the quotation from Antonin Scalia. In many cases, the court has shown a deference to psychiatry, determining that due process need not always include a judicial review of doctors' decisions, but, in others, has required oversight from the court, depending on the individual right and the state interest at stake in the particular case. This tension between the need for psychiatry in the courts, and its limits, has manifest most prominently in discussions of psychiatric diagnosis, civil commitment, and predictions of dangerousness.

Debate rages within the medical profession as to whether "alcoholism" is a separate "disease" in any meaningful biochemical, physiological or psychological sense, or whether it represents one peculiar manifestation in some individuals of underlying psychiatric disorders.[41]

Having ruled in *Robinson v. California*[42] that an individual could not be punished criminally for the status of being a drug addict, in *Powell v. Texas*[41] the court considered whether or not Leroy Powell should likewise not be held responsible for being drunk in public because he suffered from alcoholism. Two related but distinct disputes regarding the uncertainty of psychiatric diagnosis emerged: first, how the medical community defined addiction; and second, to what extent could medicine determine the extent to which addiction overrode an individual's autonomy?

Assuming that that term can be given a reasonably precise content and that the 'mentally ill' can be identified with reasonable accuracy, there is still no constitutional basis for confining such persons involuntarily if they are dangerous to no one and can live safely in freedom.[2]

The case of *O'Connor vs. Donaldson*[2] is a landmark case for many reasons, but its perspective with regards to uncertainty about psychiatric diagnosis represents a pivot point, linking that uncertainty to psychiatric predictions of dangerousness, with which the *O'Connor* court coupled, via the Fourteenth Amendment, justification for civil commitment. The case of *Addington v. Texas*[7] directly addresses the tension between the court's reliance on and need for psychiatric expert testimony and its inherent uncertainty with regards to providing adequate due process: "Given the lack of certainty and the fallibility of psychiatric diagnosis, there is a serious question as to whether a state could ever prove beyond a reasonable doubt that an individual is both mentally ill and likely to be dangerous. . . The subtleties and nuances of psychiatric diagnosis render certainties virtually beyond reach in most situations."[7]

The psychiatric debate, therefore, helps to inform the law by setting the bounds of what is reasonable, but it cannot here decide just how States must write their laws within those bounds.[17]

Debates about how psychiatry defines mental illness, and its relevance, if any, resurface in cases such as *Kansas v. Hendricks*,[17] where the court debates whether or not the "mental abnormality" required to classify a person as a sexually violent predator in *Kansas* maps onto medical definitions of mental disorders. The court undergoes a similar analysis in *Foucha v. Louisiana*,[43] considering the meaning of "antisocial personality" in the context of continued confinement for a man found not guilty by reason of insanity. The courts rely on the precedents set down in *O'Connor*[2] and *Addington*[7] regarding mental illness, dangerousness, and civil commitment, and therefore must wrestle with whether or not these kinds of deviant behavior fit that mold.

Neither petitioner nor the Association suggests that psychiatrists are always wrong with respect to future dangerousness, only most of the time.

The suggestion that no psychiatrist's testimony may be presented with respect to a defendant's future dangerousness is somewhat like asking us to disinvent the wheel.[44]

This tension comes full circle in *Barefoot v. Estelle*,[44] in which Mr. Barefoot, attempting to appeal his death sentence, argues that psychiatric predictions of dangerousness are so unreliable that they ought never be admitted, at least in the context of capital sentencing. The majority decides that the jury can be trusted to determine the reliability of psychiatric predictions of dangerousness. However, the dissent is careful to dissect out death penalty cases from other areas of law in which psychiatric testimony may be sufficiently reliable, though in capital cases it is not: "In the present state of psychiatric knowledge, this is too much for me. In a capital case, the specious testimony of a psychiatrist, colored in the eyes of an impressionable jury by the inevitable untouchability of a medical specialist's words, equates with death itself."

Perhaps because there often is no single, accurate psychiatric conclusion on legal insanity in a given case, juries remain the primary factfinders on this issue, and they must resolve differences in opinion within the psychiatric profession on the basis of the evidence offered by each party.[45]

Barefoot firmly establishes a role for psychiatrists in determinations of dangerousness, warts and all, even when the stakes are highest, in terms of meeting out the death penalty. To this end, in *Ake v. Oklahoma*[45] the U.S. Supreme Court, consistent with *Barefoot*, decides that despite psychiatry's uncertainties, indigent defendants contemplating an insanity defense are entitled to an expert examiner at the state's expense.

Due process has never been thought to require that the neutral and detached trier of fact be law trained or a judicial or administrative officer. Surely, this is the case as to medical decisions, for "neither judges nor administrative hearing officers are better qualified than psychiatrists to render psychiatric judgments."[24]

In determining whether the State has met its obligations in these respects, decisions made by the appropriate professional are entitled to a presumption of correctness. Such a presumption is necessary to enable institutions of this type— often, unfortunately, overcrowded and understaffed—to continue to function.[22]

In other contexts, however, the Court has shown more deference to psychiatry. In *Parham v. JR*,[24] the U.S. Supreme Court held that an independent evaluation by a staff psychiatrist provided adequate due process for a minor's liberty interest in avoiding civil commitment, and that a judicial hearing was not required. Similarly, in *Youngberg v. Romeo*,[22] the court determined that while psychiatric inpatients had a liberty interest to avoid restraint and seclusion, the judgment of professionals provided adequate due process, in the setting of managing the safety of hospital.

Variations in the definitions of and deference to both liberty and psychiatry are but two of the many tributaries that may be followed, flowing from an in-depth study of landmark cases. That they were the themes most frequently found in our study, we suggest, reflects the importance, of autonomy in the history and identity of the United States. As discussed, all of the applications of liberty in our cases are in some way a manifestation of autonomy, the loss of which is often defined as a constitutional issue.

The changing views of psychiatry may reflect, in part, whether the courts see psychiatry as promoting, or undermining, autonomy. Does medication, for example, increase autonomy or constrain choice and action? The courts' views also reflect differences within the psychiatric community itself, from an optimistic view of psychoanalytic cure to pessimistic concern about the limits of psychopharmacology. The optimism with regards to advances in psychoanalytic insight one finds in *Durham v. U.S.*,[46] for example, which Judge Bazelon uses to open the flood gates of psychiatric opinion into the insanity defense via the product rule, stands in stark contrast to the laborious descriptions of the many side effects of antipsychotic medications in cases such as *State v. Perry*,[47] *Riggins v. Nevada*,[19] and *Rogers v. Commissioner*.[34] The courts' ambivalence, particularly in the 1980s, is not entirely dissociated from conversations within psychiatry at the time about the relative benefits of medication and talk therapy, that is, whether medication cures or merely suppresses symptoms of mental illness (also reflected in the nomenclature for the concerning antipsychotics, "major tranquilizers"). As noted earlier, however, in later cases the Court shows a greater willingness to allow physicians to make clinical decisions without court oversight.

While this may reflect a greater appreciation for the science of mental illness and potential of mental health treatment, another explanatory cross-current that becomes evident through the chronological landmark case review is the changing political landscape, in which more conservative courts are less inclined to support an expansive definition of liberty, less inclined to require, therefore, court oversight, less inclined to set policy from the bench, more inclined to defer to the states and localities, and more inclined to defer to the traditional authority of the professionals. This, then, is yet another important theme in landmark case study, enhancing appreciation for the history of mental health and forensic psychiatry and expanding understanding of the ever-changing intersection between law and psychiatry.

It is a foundational principle of training in forensic psychiatry that whether practicing clinical care or performing forensic evaluations, an understanding of the relevant law is critical to appropriate assessment and decision making. This necessary competency is enhanced when one understands how the law thinks and evolves. As demonstrated earlier, tracing the index cases (e.g., *Jackson* and *Addington*) through subsequent landmark cases, sociopolitical themes and legal principles emerge. As important as the specific holdings in mental health law are to clinical and forensic practice, a stand-alone Landmark Case seminar allows broader themes and principles to be mined (of which liberty and uncertainty about psychiatry are but two examples); and in this model, the issue of mental illness or a behavioral health disorder not *the* point, but rather just the starting point.

REFERENCES

1. American Academy of Psychiatry the Law. *Landmark Cases 2014.* www.aapl.org/landmark- cases.
2. O'Connor v. Donaldson, 422 U.S. 563 (1975).
3. Accreditation Council for Graduate Medical Education. ACGME Program Requirements for Graduate Medical Education in Forensic Psychiatry. https://www.acgme.org/Portals/0/PFAssets/ProgramRequirements/406_forensic_psych_2016_1- YR.pdf.
4. Appelbaum, P. (1994). *Almost a revolution.* New York: Oxford University Press.
5. Rotter, M., & Forman, H. (2017). The case for landmark cases. In R. Rosner & C. Scott (Eds.), *Principles and practice of forensic psychiatry* (3rd ed., xxx–xxx). Boca Raton, FL: Taylor and Francis Group.
6. Jackson v. Indiana, 406 U.S. 715, 92 S.Ct. 1845 (1972).
7. Addington v. Texas, 441 U.S. 418, 99 S.Ct. 1804 (1979).
8. Cooper v. Oklahoma, 571 U.S. 348 (1996).
9. Godinez v. Moran, 509 U.S. 162 (1993).
10. Drope v. Missouri, 420 U.S. 162 (1975).
11. Zinermon v. Burch, 494 U.S. 113, 110 S.Ct. 975 (1990).
12. Washington v. Harper, 494 U.S. 210, 110 S.Ct. 1028 (1990).
13. Fasulo v. Arafeh, 378 A.2d 553 (1977).
14. In re Young, 857 P.2d. 989 (1993).
15. Vitek v. Jones, 445 U.S 480, 100 S.Ct. 1254 (1980).
16. Cruzan v. Director, Missouri DMH, 497 U.S 261, 110 S.Ct. 2841 (1990).
17. Kansas v. Hendricks, 521 U.S. 346 (1997).
18. Jones v. U.S., 463 U.S. 354, 103 S.Ct. 3043 (1983)
19. Riggins v. Nevada, 504 U.S. 127, 112 S.Ct. 1810 (1992).
20. Allen v. Illinois, 478 U.S. 364, 106 S.Ct. 2988 (1986).
21. Kansas v. Crane, 534 U.S. 407, 122 S.Ct. 867 (2002).
22. Youngberg v. Romeo, 457 U.S. 307, 102 S.Ct. 2452 (1982).
23. Rennie v. Klein, 720 F.2d 266 (1983).
24. Parham v. JR, 442 U.S. 584, 99 S.Ct. 2493 (1979).
25. In re Richardson, 481 A.2d 473 (1984).
26. Ford v. Wainwright, 477 U.S. 399, 106 S.Ct. 2595 (1986).
27. http://constitution.findlaw.com/amendment14.html.
28. http://www.ushistory.org/DECLARATION/document/.

29. Allgeyer v. Louisiana, 165 U.S. 578 (1897).
30. Humphrey v. Cady, 405 U.S. 504 (1972).
31. Baxstrom v. Herold, 383 U.S. 107, 86 S.Ct. 760 (1966).
32. Clites v. Iowa, 322 N.W. 2d 917 (Iowa Ct. App. 1982).
33. DeShaney v. Winnebago County Dept. of Social Services, 489 U.S. 189, 109 S.Ct. 998 (1989).
34. Rogers v. Commissioner of Dept. of Mental Health, 390 Mass. 489, 458 N.E.2d 308 (1983).
35. Estelle v. Gamble, 429 U.S. 97, 97 S.Ct. 285 (1976).
36. Superintendent of Belchertown State School v. Saikewicz, 370 N.E.2d 417 (1977).
37. Washington v. Glucksberg, 521 U.S. 702 (1997).
38. Vacco v. Quill, 521 U.S. 793 (1997).
39. Chodoff, P. (1976). The case for involuntary hospitalization of the mentally ill. *American Journal of Psychiatry, 133*(5), 496–501.
40. Jaffee v. Redmond, 518 US. 1 (1996).
41. Powell v. Texas, 392 U.S. 514, 88 S.Ct. 2145 (1968).
42. Robinson v. California, 370 U.S. 660, 82 S.Ct. 1417 (1962).
43. Foucha v. Louisiana, 504 U.S. 71 (1992).
44. Barefoot v. Estelle, 463 U.S. 880, 103 S.Ct. 3383 (1983).
45. Ake v. Oklahoma, 470 U.S. 68, 105 S.Ct. 1087 (1985).
46. Durham v. U.S., 94 U.S. App. D.C. 228, 214 F.2d 862 (1954).
47. State v. Perry, 610 So.2d 746 (1992).

SECTION I

Mental Health Practice Guidelines

CHAPTER 1

cᴧɔ

Confidentiality and Privilege

S. SHANE KONRAD AND ERAKA BATH

IN RE LIFSCHUTZ, 467 P.2D 557 (1970)

Link to case: https://scocal.stanford.edu/opinion/re-lifschutz-22784

Question: Can a psychiatrist assert privilege for information gathered in the course of treatment, when the patient has waived privilege?

Answer: No.

Joseph Housek was in treatment with his psychiatrist, Dr. Joseph Lifschutz, 10 years prior to filing a civil lawsuit in a California court for an alleged assault by a high school student. Mr. Housek claimed mental and emotional distress. The student defendant's attorney found out about this prior treatment and subpoenaed Dr. Lifschutz and his records. Dr. Lifschutz appeared in court as a witness but refused to provide medical records or give testimony about Mr. Housek's treatment. The court ordered Dr. Lifschutz to testify based on the California statutory patient-litigant exception under which Mr. Housek had waived his privacy privilege by initiating the lawsuit, asking for damages for pain and suffering, and making his emotional state an issue. Dr. Lifschutz was found in contempt and jailed for several days. Dr. Lifschutz filed for habeas corpus. Dr. Lifschutz claimed that the court order was invalid as unconstitutionally infringing on his personal right of privacy, his right to effectively practice his profession, the constitutional privacy rights of his patients, and his right to equal protection, comparing his role as psychotherapist to that of the clergy. The California Supreme Court confirmed the contempt of court finding, and the writ of habeas corpus was denied. The court found that the need for confidentiality in psychotherapy must be balanced with society's need for determining the truth. Most important, the Court affirmed that the patient, not the therapist, had the right to privacy, and therefore the exclusive ability to waive that right. The Court cited the constitutional protection of the practice of religion, as distinct from psychotherapy, in denying Lifschutz' equal protection claim.

DOE V. ROE, 93. MISC. 2D 201 (1977)

Link to case: http://scholar.google.com/scholar_case?
case=4446229919103114898

Question: Is patient confidentiality violated by the publication of information, without informed consent, obtained during psychiatric treatment?

Answer: Yes.

Jane Doe (a pseudonym) sued her former psychiatrist, Dr. Jane Roe (also a pseudonym), and Dr. Roe's psychologist husband for damages, alleging that they unlawfully violated her privacy by publishing a book that included information obtained during Ms. Doe's couples psychotherapy sessions. The book was released years after the treatment and included "verbatim and extensively the patient's thoughts, feelings, emotions, fantasies, and biographies." Ms. Doe requested to have the publication stopped. The trial court, without a jury, held that the publication should be stopped, and Ms. Doe was awarded $20,000 in compensatory damages. The New York State Supreme Court found that licensing regulations and professional ethical codes required that information shared in the physician–patient relationship be kept confidential. The court noted that "patients could only reveal their most intimate and socially unacceptable instincts and urges, immature wishes, and perverse sexual thoughts in an atmosphere of unusual trust."

The court rejected Dr. Roe's rebuttals that she had obtained oral consent from Ms. Doe, that the book contributed to scientific knowledge, and that she had adequately disguised Ms. Doe's identity. The court also found that privacy rights of patients limited free speech rights. The court rejected punitive damages because Dr. Roe's actions were not willful, malicious, or wanton as required by law but "merely stupid." Of note, Dr. Roe's husband was also held liable. Even though he was not Ms. Doe's psychiatrist, he helped to write, promote and distribute the book and was, therefore, a "willing violator of the patient's rights."

WHALEN V. ROE, 429 U.S. 589 (1977)

Link to case: http://caselaw.lp.findlaw.com/scripts/getcase.pl?navby=case&
court=us&vol=429&page=589

Question: Can a state constitutionally collect personal information about
patients who are receiving prescriptions for narcotics?

Answer: Yes.

In 1972, the New York state legislature enacted the New York State
Controlled Substances Act because of concern that certain prescription
drugs were being unlawfully diverted. The act required doctors to fill out,
and submit to the Department of Health, forms for Schedule II prescription drugs, which included patients' personal information such as the
patient's name, age, and address. Physicians and patients brought an action
challenging the constitutionality of this statute. Even though the statute
prohibited public disclosure of the patient's identity, the plaintiffs voiced
concern about the privacy of patients who had their personal information
stored in a centralized computer. The district court found the New York
law unconstitutional, stating that some patients may decline necessary
medications out of concern that misuse of the computerized data could
cause them to be stigmatized as "drug addicts." The U.S. Supreme Court
heard the case on appeal and reversed the district court decision. The Court
held, noting in part the "remote possibility" of potential abuse of the data
collected, the requirements of the act adequately addressed the constitutionally based "zone of privacy" as well as the rights and liberties protected
by the Fourteenth Amendment.

IN RE SUBPOENA SERVED UPON ZUNIGA, 714 F.2D 632 (1983)

Link to case: http://www.leagle.com/decision/19831346714F2d632_
11238

Question: Can a psychotherapist's refusal to respond to a grand jury subpoena lead to a ruling of contempt?

Answer: Yes.

In a case investigating insurance fraud, the grand jury for the Eastern District
of Michigan issued a subpoena commanding a psychiatrist, Dr. Jorge Zuniga,
to appear before the grand jury and produce the following records: (1)

redacted copies of patient files indicating patient name, date of service, type of psychotherapy session rendered (i.e., full, half, brief), and amount billed; (2) original ledger cards for patients; and (3) originals of any intraoffice forms in support of services rendered and date thereof. Dr. Zuniga refused to produce these records and filed a motion in the district court to quash the subpoena. He was found in civil contempt and ordered into custody of the U.S. Marshal Service pending the outcome of the appeal. The U.S. Court of Appeals for the Sixth Circuit affirmed and held that federal rules of evidence include a recognition of psychotherapist–patient privilege, but the limited patient identification information Dr. Zuniga was required to release to the court was not protected by the privilege, both because of the limited nature of disclosure and because the patient's had implicitly waived identification as privileged when they allowed disclosure to Blue Cross for insurance purposes. The appellate court also found that release of this information to the grand jury was not a violation of patients' privacy rights, given the "veil of secrecy" in grand jury proceedings. The court also found that Dr. Zuniga could not invoke his Fifth Amendment privilege against self-incrimination to defend his refusal to release records because he was incorporated and not functioning as a private individual in this situation.

STATE V. ANDRING, 342 N.W.2D 128 (1984)

Link to case: http://scholar.google.com/scholar_case?
case=18146708613969658932

Question: Does the scope of the physician–patient privilege extend to group therapy?

Answer: Yes.

David Andring had been criminally charged in Minnesota for sexual misconduct with his 10-year-old stepdaughter and 11-year-old niece. While awaiting trial, he voluntarily entered a treatment facility, where he received individual and group therapy for alcohol treatment. He openly disclosed the sexual abuse in both individual and group therapy settings. When prosecutors became aware of his treatment, they moved to obtain and present his treatment records as evidence. While the trial court denied the admittance of his intake and individual therapy records, it did permit release of his group therapy records. Mr. Andring appealed and argued that the Federal Comprehensive Alcohol Abuse and Alcoholism Prevention, Treatment and Rehabilitation Act Amendments of 1974 ("federal alcohol treatment act") preempted any disclosure of treatment-related information. The Supreme Court of Minnesota reversed the decision, finding that while state-mandated reported of abuse was an exception to the federal confidentiality requirements, this did not necessarily extend to all requests by the state or its prosecutors. Physician–patient privilege did, however, extend to group therapy sessions, because the third parties in the group sessions were part of the treatment process, the abuse was already known, and his group therapy session records were not necessary to proceed with the criminal prosecution. The court noted that violation of physician–patient privilege from the group therapy sessions would not serve to further protect the children.

COMMONWEALTH V. KOBRIN, 479 N.E.2D 674 (1985)

Link to case: http://scholar.google.com/scholar_case?
case=18127391409676670050

Question: Can a limited set of records be subpoenaed from a psychiatrist to investigate billing fraud?

Answer: Yes.

A grand jury in Massachusetts subpoenaed complete records of patients whose cases were being investigated for alleged fraud violations of the Medicaid False Claim Act. In this particular case, 27 patients of Dr. Kennard Kobrin, a psychiatrist, objected to the disclosure of their personal medical records, citing invasion of privacy. Dr. Kobrin refused to provide the records, but a superior court judge ordered the records to be produced. Dr. Kobrin then produced "sanitized" copies of the patients' charts, citing his patients' rights to exercise their psychotherapist–patient privilege. He was held in contempt, and his records were seized. The Supreme Court of Massachusetts found that both the government's need to know and the patients' confidentiality could be accommodated. The court held that Kobrin could submit records documenting "times and lengths of patient appointments, fees, patient diagnoses, treatment plans and recommendations, and somatic therapies." This limited information would allow for a legitimate investigation. Those portions of records reflecting any patient's thoughts, feelings, impressions, or containing the substance of any psychotherapeutic dialogue, or exposing personal relationships were of no concern to legitimate investigation.

MENENDEZ V. SUPERIOR COURT, 834 P.2D 786 (1992)

Link to case: http://scholar.google.com/scholar_case?
case=11801048403762594860

Question: Does the psychotherapist–patient privilege apply to treatment records regarding dangerousness?

Answer: No.

In this highly publicized case, brothers Erik and Lyle Menendez were charged with murdering their parents. A magistrate in the Municipal Court of the Beverly Hills Judicial District of Los Angeles County issued a search warrant authorizing a search of the office and residence of Leon Jerome Oziel, PhD (a clinical psychologist who was Erik and Lyle's psychotherapist), and seizure of specified items if found therein, including audiotape recordings containing information relating to the killings. The brothers filed a petition in support of Dr. Oziel, who claimed that audiotapes he made of his notes and of sessions with the Menendez brothers were covered by psychotherapist–patient privilege. On several tapes there was documentation of the brothers' threats of harm to Dr. Oziel, and on others there were threats to his lover and his wife. A California superior court and then the California Supreme Court found that some of the audiotapes could be disclosed. The California Supreme Court found that the tapes which included information disclosed to the patients' parents met the "dangerous person" exception to the therapist–patient privilege; that is, they contained information indicating a patient is dangerous and disclosure of dangerousness was necessary to prevent harm. The "dangerous person" exception requires that the psychotherapist have reasonable cause for belief of dangerousness. It does not demand that the patient must be dangerous to a person other than the psychotherapist—although in this case the patients were.

JAFFEE V. REDMOND, 518 U.S. 1 (1996)

Link to case: http://caselaw.lp.findlaw.com/scripts/getcase.pl?navby=case&court=us&vol=518&page=1

Question: Should federal courts identify a psychotherapist–patient privilege?

Answer: Yes.

Mary Lu Redmond was the first police officer to respond to a "fight in progress" call at an apartment complex. According to Redmond, Ricky Allen was brandishing a knife when he came out of the apartment and disregarded her repeated commands to drop the weapon. Redmond shot and killed Allen when she believed he was about to stab the man he was chasing. Carrie Jaffee was the special administrator of Allen's estate and filed suit in federal district court alleging that Redmond had violated Allen's constitutional rights by using excessive force. After this traumatic event, Redmond participated in about 50 counseling sessions with Karen Beyer, a licensed clinical social worker. Beyer and Redmond refused requests to share information discussed in their sessions with the court. They asserted that this information was protected against involuntary disclosure by a psychotherapist–patient privilege. The district judge rejected this argument and advised the jury that Beyer's refusal to turn over her notes had no "legal justification," and the jury could presume that the records were unfavorable to Redmond. The U.S. Court of Appeals for the Seventh Circuit reversed and remanded for a new trial. The court concluded that "reason and experience," the touchstones for acceptance of a privilege under Rule 501 of the Federal Rules of Evidence, compelled recognition of a psychotherapist–patient privilege. "Reason tells us that psychotherapists and patients share a unique relationship, in which the ability to communicate freely without the fear of public disclosure is the key to successful treatment." As to experience, the court observed that all 50 states have adopted some form of the psychotherapist–patient privilege. The U.S. Supreme Court affirmed the appellate court ruling, explicitly including social workers within the definition of psychotherapists.

CHAPTER 2

❧

Informed Consent

GREGORY DAVIS

NATANSON V. KLINE, 350 P.2D 1093 (1960)

Link to case: http://scholar.google.com/scholar_case?
case=1590825446079418783

Question: Is informed consent required for nonnegligent physician care?

Answer: Yes.

Irma Natanson sustained burns from cobalt radiation therapy as part of her treatment for breast cancer. She filed a malpractice suit against her radiologist, Dr. Kline, claiming that she was not adequately informed of the risks of treatment beforehand. Although the trial court found that the doctor was not negligent, upon appeal, the Kansas Supreme Court found that the trial court committed error in not specifically instructing the jury with regard to the amount of disclosure sufficient for a physician to obtain informed consent. According to the appellate court, elements required for informed consent include the nature of the illness, the proposed treatment, alternative treatment, the probability of success, and the risks involved. Ms. Natanson requested an instruction to the jury that a physician had a duty to make a full disclosure to the patient of all matters within his knowledge affecting the interests of the patient. The Kansas Supreme Court found that the requested instruction was too broad, stating that a physician's duty is limited to disclosures that a "reasonable medical practitioner" would make under similar circumstances. This standard assumes that a consensus exists within the medical community and allows the physician to use his or her medical judgment.

CANTERBURY V. SPENCE, 464 F.2D 772 (1972)

Link to case: http://scholar.google.com/scholar_case?
case=16106013819601769055

Question: Can a physician be liable for malpractice if he or she fails to disclose severe, although rare, risks inherent in a medical procedure?

Answer: Yes.

Jerry Canterbury underwent a laminectomy performed by Dr. Spence as part of an evaluation of his back pain. The day after the surgery, Mr. Canterbury fell from his unattended hospital bed, leading to paraplegia and incontinence. He filed suit for negligence, alleging in part that he was not informed of the 1% risk of paralysis that Dr. Spence testified would be anticipated with a laminectomy. Dr. Spence said that communication of risk of paralysis was not good medical practice because it might deter patients from undergoing needed surgery. After an initial finding for Dr. Spence, the case was brought before the District of Columbia Court of Appeals, which reversed and elaborated on the scope of the disclosure requirement necessary for informed consent. The court reasoned that a professional medical standard such as described in *Natanson v. Kline* is at odds with a patient's prerogative to decide on a proposed treatment. In its view, the patient's autonomy shapes the boundaries of disclosure. Based on medical training and experience, the court said, a physician can sense how much an average, reasonable patient would want to know. The court defined the standard for disclosure as being based on what a "reasonable person" would find material to decision making, including serious, but rare, risks. It noted two exceptions as an incapacitated person in an emergency situation and, in rare instances, if disclosure itself may do harm.

KAIMOWITZ V. DEPARTMENT OF MENTAL HEALTH FOR THE STATE OF MICHIGAN, NO. 73-19434-AW, MICH. CIR. CT., WAYNE CO. (1973)

Link to case: http://psychrights.org/Research/Legal/InformedConsent/
KaimowitzvMichDeptMH%28MichCir1973%29.pdf

Question: Does involuntary commitment to a state psychiatric facility preclude providing adequate informed consent for experimental psychosurgery?

Answer: Yes.

John Doe had been committed to the Ionia State hospital in 1955 under a criminal sexual psychopathy law in Michigan. Mr. Doe provided informed consent to participate in a study of uncontrolled aggression. The study utilized experimental techniques and compared amygdaloid surgery to administration of the drug cyproterone. A third party, Mr. Kaimowitz, filed a writ of habeas corpus alleging that Mr. Doe was being illegally detained for surgery. The court directed Mr. Doe's release but also opined about the legality of the consent process. The court reasoned that when compared with accepted treatments, experimental psychosurgery could have substantial risk with no known benefits. It noted that informed consent should be closely scrutinized for procedures with a high risk-to-benefit ratio and should be competent, knowing, and voluntary—none of which were possible, given the inherently coercive nature of his confinement and the lack of factual support for the procedure. The court referenced the Nuremberg Code statement that experimental subjects should be able to exercise free power of choice without force, deceit, duress, or coercion. In addition, the court also found support for its decision in the constitutional rights of freedom of speech and privacy. The court concluded that involuntarily confined patients, such as Mr. Doe in a state hospital, live in an "inherently coercive" situation that makes it impossible to give voluntary consent for a risky procedure. Of note, the ruling applied only to experimental psychosurgery; the court held that an involuntarily detained mental patient could possibly give adequate consent for accepted medical procedures.

TRUMAN V. THOMAS, 611 P.2D 902 (1980)

Link to case: http://scholar.google.com/scholar_case?
case=4583670149937548076

Question: Can a physician be found liable for failing to inform a patient of the consequences of not getting a recommended medical test?

Answer: Yes.

Rena Truman was a 30-year-old woman who died after having been diagnosed with late-stage cervical cancer. She had not had a Pap smear for 5 years despite regular visits to her family practitioner, Dr. Claude Thomas. Following her death, her two children sued Dr. Thomas for malpractice. At trial, the judge refused to permit jury instruction that a physician has a duty to disclose all relevant information, including the risk of refusing procedures. The jury found in favor of Dr. Thomas, but upon appeal the Supreme Court of California reversed the trial court decision, citing judicial error. The court considered whether the physician breached his duty when he did not inform Mrs. Truman of the risk of failing to receive a Pap smear. Dr. Thomas contended that patients who reject their physician's advice should shoulder the burden of possible consequences. He also argued that he did not have a duty because the danger was remote and commonly known. The court explained that a patient is dependent on the physician for information because the physician has a greater degree of specialized medical knowledge. The court noted that despite being remote, the risk was death, and there was no evidence that the risk was commonly known. The court held that all material information that a reasonable person would want to know was relevant, including the risk of refusing a test. However, the court also noted that to find proximate cause, the jury would have to find that, but for the lack of disclosure, the plaintiff would not have refused the procedure.

CLITES V. IOWA, 322 N.W.2D 917 (1982)

Link to case: http://ia.findacase.com/research/wfrmDocViewer.aspx/xq/fac.19820629_0042174.IA.htm/qx

Question: Can failure to obtain informed consent for antipsychotic medication be grounds for malpractice?

Answer: Yes.

Timothy Clites was a man with mental retardation who was placed in restraints and received a variety of antipsychotic medications for aggressive behavior while admitted to a state-operated residential facility. Mr. Clites developed tardive dyskinesia after 5 years of treatment. His father sued for a violation of civil rights and damages from negligence. The trial court found for Mr. Clites, citing a lack of evidence of aggression, no regular evaluation by a physician for 3 years, no consultation for tardive dyskinesia, use of medications and restraints as a convenience, and lack of informed consent. The Iowa Court of Appeals affirmed the decision and underscored the informed consent required for administration of antipsychotic medication. The court reasoned that the concept of a right to privacy implied an underlying right to think and decide for oneself. Absent an emergency situation, a competent patient has a fundamental right to decide to be left alone without medications. The court concluded that there is a recognized standard that requires informed consent prior to administration of antipsychotic medication. As part of informed consent, a physician has a duty to make a reasonable disclosure of the nature and probable consequences of the recommended treatment.

ZINERMON V. BURCH, 494 U.S. 113 (1990)

Link to case: http://scholar.google.com/scholar_case?
case=17065115765946990987

Question: Can an incompetent individual consent to voluntary hospitalization?

Answer: No.

Darrell Burch was admitted to a Florida state mental hospital in 1981 after being found wandering on a highway in Tallahassee while hallucinating, telling officials he was "in heaven." He signed voluntary admission forms despite never having been evaluated for capacity. Voluntary admission in Florida required "express and informed consent." He later brought a civil rights action claiming that the hospital had deprived him of liberty without due process as afforded by the Fourteenth Amendment. Mr. Burch alleged that state law was violated because the hospital should have known that he was incompetent to give informed consent to sign voluntary forms; hence, he was entitled to procedural safeguards of an involuntary admission. The case was initially dismissed, on the basis that while he was deprived of liberty, postdeprivation remedy was not required. However, the U.S. Supreme Court ultimately agreed with Mr. Burch. It held that because the hospital's staff had authority to deprive persons of liberty, the Constitution imposed on them the state's duty to provide procedural protections. The Court contended that it was foreseeable that a person requesting treatment for mental illness might not be capable of informed consent, which should be specifically assessed at the time of admission. The state's violation of the duty to investigate the patient's competence was "fully predictable" and not a "random, unauthorized" violation of law as the state contended. Therefore, without deciding the merits of Zinermon's specific case, the Court found that predeprivation due process guarantees were theoretically possible, postdeprivation remedy should be available, and Zinermon, at least, had stated a triable claim.

CHAPTER 3

༄

Duty to Protect

ANDREW M. KOPELMAN

TARASOFF V. REGENTS, 551 P.2D 334 (1976)

Link to case: https://scocal.stanford.edu/opinion/tarasoff-v-regents-university-california-30278

Question: Is there a therapist duty to protect a third party from a dangerous patient?

Answer: Yes.

The parents of Tatiana Tarasoff sued the University of California and the psychologist working for its student health clinic after a patient in this clinic, Mr. Prosenjit Poddar, murdered Ms. Tarasoff. Mr. Poddar had confided to his psychologist his intention to kill Ms. Tarasoff, who was readily identifiable by Mr. Poddar's description. While the doctor and clinic did take some steps to contain the risk that Mr. Poddar represented, such as notifying the campus police, no one directly warned Ms. Tarasoff. The trial court found that the psychologist could not be held directly liable for failing to successfully hospitalize Mr. Poddar; the appeals court agreed, and a further appeal was made to the California Supreme Court. The doctors argued that they did not necessarily have a duty to someone other than their identified patient, that dangerousness was too difficult to predict, and that the nature of psychotherapeutic practice required protection of patient confidentiality. That court reversed the appellate decision in 1974 and found that therapists have a duty to *warn* individuals threatened by patients (known as *Tarasoff* I). In light of unusual protest about this decision, including from psychiatrists, the California Supreme Court agreed to hear the case again in 1976 (*Tarasoff*

II). Beginning its analysis with the common law assumption that no one owed a duty to control the conduct of another, the court held that the special relationship between a psychotherapist and a patient created a duty to *protect* others from an identifiably dangerous patient based on the logic of foreseeability. The court majority relied heavily on precedents involving contagious diseases to formulate this notion. "When a therapist determines, or pursuant to the standards of his profession should determine, that his patient presents a serious danger of violence to another," the psychotherapist has a duty to "exercise reasonable care" in protecting the potential victim, including possibly—but not necessarily—directly warning the potential victim. The court disagreed with defendant's arguments regarding the potential effects on clinical practice and the inability of clinicians to predict violence. As the court maintained, "The protective privilege [i.e., confidentiality] ends where the public peril begins."

LIPARI V. SEARS, 497 F. SUPP. 1985 (1980)

Link to case: http://scholar.google.com/scholar_case?case=1021277736768084136

Question: Does a psychiatrist's duty to protect third parties extend to foreseeable, but unidentified, third parties?

Answer: Yes.

Ruth Ann Lipari sued Sears & Roebuck Co. after she was shot and her husband was killed by Ulysses Cribbs in a crowded nightclub in Omaha, Nebraska. Mr. Cribbs had purchased the shotgun at Sears. Mr. Cribbs had previously been committed to a Veterans Administration (VA) psychiatric hospital and subsequently treated as a VA outpatient approximately 1 month before the shooting. Mrs. Lipari argued that Sears should not have sold a gun to someone who was known to be "mentally defective." Sears in turn filed a third-party suit under the Federal Torts Claim Act, alleging that the VA hospital's negligent care of Mr. Cribbs was the proximate cause for the shooting injury and death. Mrs. Lipari then sued the U.S. government as well. The government petitioned the Nebraska Supreme Court for a summary motion dismissing these claims. In rejecting the government's position, the Nebraska court extended the reasoning of *Tarasoff* (California) to the state of Nebraska. The court affirmed that the special relationship between a psychotherapist and a patient imposed an affirmative duty to protect third parties from potentially dangerous patients. In acknowledging the technical difficulties related to violence prediction, the court explained that psychiatrists were not responsible for all acts of dangerous patients.

Rather, the liability from a failure in the duty to protect arose from negligent practice that did not meet the professional standard of "due care." The victims need not be readily identifiable as was the case in *Tarasoff*, but instead belong to a "class of persons" who could be "reasonably foreseen" to be harmed by the dangerous patient.

PETERSEN V. WASHINGTON, 671 P.2D 230 (1983)

Link to case: http://www.leagle.com/decision/1983521100Wn2d421_1482

Question: Does a psychiatrist's duty to third parties include protecting foreseeable victims from potential danger caused by a patient's noncompliance with medication?

Answer: Yes.

Cynthia Petersen sued the State of Washington after being injured in a motor vehicle accident involving a driver, Larry Knox, who ran a red light while under the influence of drugs. Mr. Knox had been released from a state psychiatric hospital only 5 days prior. Dr. Alva Miller, Mr. Knox's psychiatrist, argued that Mr. Knox had "recovered" at the time of his discharge. The trial court allowed rebuttal evidence about Mr. Knox's previous psychotic presentations to hospitals and subsequent arrests. A jury found that Dr. Miller negligently treated Mr. Knox by failing to seek further involuntary confinement at the time of discharge, or other attempts to address what Dr. Miller admitted was the likelihood of nonadherence to medication and recurrent drug use; and that this negligence was the proximate cause of Ms. Petersen injuries. On appeal, the Supreme Court of Washington affirmed the verdict, agreeing that the special relationship between a psychiatrist and a patient created a third-party duty to protect anyone who might "foreseeably be endangered" by Mr. Knox's illness, including his propensity to stop medication and return to abusing PCP. The court rejected the state's claim that it was not liable for negligence because Dr. Miller was performing a "discretionary activity of government" (i.e., performing an activity related to basic governmental policy) in completing a risk assessment.

JABLONSKI V. U.S., 712 F.2D 391 (1983)

Link to case: http://scholar.google.com/scholar_case?
case=1021277736768084136

Question: Is a psychiatrist required to protect a foreseeable victim in the absence of a specific threat?

Answer: Yes.

Philip Jablonski received an outpatient evaluation at the Loma Linda VA hospital after threatening Melinda Kimball's mother. Diagnosing the patient with "antisocial personality," the psychiatrist, Dr. Kopytoff, did not make an effort to obtain Mr. Jablonski's medical records, which revealed the patient had suffered from schizophrenia and had tried to kill his previous wife on multiple occasions. Mr. Jablonski returned for another evaluation with Dr. Kopiloff's supervisor, but he was not hospitalized. Three days later he killed Ms. Kimball. Meghan Jablonski, Ms. Kimball's daughter, sued the U.S. government for malpractice, claiming that Dr. Kopiloff had not adequately incorporated information from the police into his assessment, had not pursued the patient's medical record, and had not specifically warned Ms. Kimball that she was at risk. The district court agreed. On appeal, the Ninth Circuit Court of Appeals affirmed the decision, rejecting the government's claim that the treating psychiatrist was subject to immunity under the Federal Torts Claim Act. The court also concluded that although Mr. Jablonski had never specifically voiced threats to Dr. Kopiloff related to Ms. Kimball, had he reviewed past medical records, she could have been clearly identified and warned as the likely victim based on Mr. Jablonski's history of domestic abuse when psychotic in the past. Finally, the court dismissed the lack of proximate cause, noting that although dangers to Ms. Kimball had been discussed with her by various parties, along with recommendations to keep her distance, she was not specifically warned by Dr. Kopiloff.

NAIDU V. LAIRD, 539 A.2D 1064 (1988)

Link to case: http://scholar.google.com/scholar_case? case=10922092048534834221

Question: Does a psychiatrist have a duty to protect the public from a dangerous former patient?

Answer: Yes.

Ann Laird sued Dr. Venkataramana Naidu of Delaware State Hospital (DSH) after Mrs. Laird's husband was killed in a motor vehicle accident caused by a recent patient of DSH, Hilton Putney. Mr. Putney had been discharged from DSH by Dr. Naidu 5 months prior after submitting a sign-out letter during a voluntary hospitalization. A jury found that Dr. Naidu's decision to discharge the patient without an adequate follow-up plan and without consideration of an involuntary commitment order was an act of negligence and the proximate cause of Mr. Laird's death. The Supreme Court of Delaware affirmed, first applying *Tarasoff* logic to affirm that the special relationship between Dr. Naidu and his patient created a third-party "broad-based obligation to protect the public from potentially violent patients." The court dismissed Dr. Naidu's claim that he was not obligated to consider Mr. Putney's psychiatric history in making an immediate assessment of dangerousness. Evidence presented at trial demonstrated that Dr. Naidu had not properly reviewed the extensive records from Mr. Putney's multiple prior hospitalizations demonstrating a history of poor medication compliance. In accepting the jury's finding of fact that Dr. Naidu's negligence was the proximate cause of Mr. Laird's death, the court also held that "temporal span" alone (i.e., more than 5 months since discharge) was not sufficient to absolve Dr. Naidu of responsibility. Finally, the court rejected Dr. Naidu's and the Delaware Psychiatric Association's arguments that the general inexactitude of dangerousness predictions prevented a case-by-case recovery from negligent psychiatric decision making, or that a verdict against Dr. Naidu might create destructive public policy in encouraging psychiatrists to avoid treating potentially violent patients or to overpredict dangerousness.

CHAPTER 4

᠅

Expert Testimony

SCOTT SOLOWAY, BRYAN C. SHELBY,
HEATHER ELLIS CUCOLO, AND JEREMY COLLEY

FRYE V. U.S., 293 F. 1013 (1923)

Link to case: http://www.law.ufl.edu/_pdf/faculty/little/topic8.pdf

Question: Is evidence acceptable in a federal criminal trial if not yet accepted by the scientific community?

Answer: No.

James Frye was convicted of murder. He appealed his conviction to the DC Circuit Court of Appeals, claiming that the lower court did not allow him to present results of the "systolic blood pressure deception test" he had undergone. His legal team argued that an expert "skilled in that particular science, art, or trade to which the question relates" could testify. The attorneys for Frye and the court recognized that no clear case law existed defining rules for the admissibility of scientific evidence. The court of appeals found that a given scientific principle, from which an expert's testimony is deduced, "must be sufficiently established to have gained general acceptance in the particular field." It ruled that "evidential force" lies somewhere between the "experimental" and "demonstrable" stages of scientific discovery. The lie detection test had not yet gained general acceptance, so the lower court's judgment was affirmed. Some states' courts (e.g., New York) still use this "Frye test" or "general acceptance" test to determine the admissibility of scientific expert testimony.

STATE V. HURD, 414 A.2D 291 (1980)

Link to case: http://scholar.google.com/scholar_case?
case=10872079423316724679

Question: Is hypnotically refreshed testimony of a crime victim that meets
certain criteria reliable such that it is admissible in New Jersey courts?

Answer: Yes.

Jane Sell was sleeping in her apartment when an assailant attacked her.
Afterward, she could not recollect the identity of her attacker. She underwent hypnosis at the suggestion of the prosecution to assist her recall. Under hypnosis, she identified her ex-husband, Paul Hurd, as the
assailant. The defense moved to suppress her hypnotically refreshed testimony under the legal theory that unreliable identification was a violation of the defendant's due process rights to a fair trial. After considering
the testimony from several experts, the trial court found that hypnotically refreshed testimony by a victim could be admissible, under the Frye
standard on a case-by-case basis, and that the state has the burden of proof
by clear and convincing evidence to establish its reliability. Furthermore,
in order to assure that the testimony is not coercive, the court adopted six
standards for admissibility: (1) sessions must be conducted by a licensed
psychiatrist or psychologist; (2) examiners involved must be independent;
(3) information obtained by law enforcement should be written; (4) facts
should be obtained from the subject before hypnosis; (5) sessions should
be videotaped; and (6) only the hypnotist and the subject should be present during the session. The court held that the testimony presented in this
case was inadmissible because it did not meet these standards. The trial
court's decision was affirmed on appeal to the New Jersey Supreme Court,
including adoption of the recommendations for admissibility standards.

PEOPLE V. SHIRLEY, 723 P.2D 1354 (1982)

Link to case: http://scholar.google.com/scholar_case?
case=6644726564566919322

Question: In California, can a witness testify after using hypnosis to refresh
his memory?

Answer: No.

Donald Shirley was accused of raping Catherine C., a woman who worked at
a bar near Camp Pendleton in California. The consistent fact pattern of the

crime involved Ms. C.'s intoxication and later sexual intercourse with Mr. Shirley. He asserted that the interaction was consensual and that he had been invited to Ms. C.'s apartment when he had met her in the bar hours prior. Ms. C. was unable to recall important details of the events and, on the eve of the trial, underwent hypnosis by a deputy district attorney with "some training" in the procedure. The trial court allowed this testimony over Mr. Shirley's objection that Ms. C.'s recollection of events under hypnosis was "manufactured evidence." There were significant differences in her pre- and posthypnosis testimony, although she was consistent in her report of at least some forced sexual activity. Dr. Donald Shafer was called by the defense as an expert on hypnosis and testified about its lack of reliability in this case. Despite this, Mr. Shirley was convicted. He appealed the decision to the Supreme Court of California. That court agreed with him and reversed the trial court finding. They expressly declined to follow the reasoning in *State v. Hurd*, ruling that even the safeguards outlined were not enough to overcome the lack of reliability of hypnotically refreshed testimony. It found that this form of evidence did not meet the *Frye* standard of general acceptance in the scientific community and was therefore inadmissible.

ROCK V. ARKANSAS, 483 U.S. 44 (1987)

Link to case: http://scholar.google.com/scholar_case?
case=4171699802405503521

Question: Does Arkansas's blanket rule barring all hypnotically refreshed testimony by a defendant violate one's constitutional right to testify on one's own behalf?

Answer: Yes.

Vickie Lorene Rock was charged with manslaughter in the death of her husband, who was found shot with a bullet wound to his chest. Ms. Rock was not able to remember the exact details of the shooting, and at the request of her attorney, she underwent hypnosis to refresh her recollection of those events. Under hypnosis, she related details of the shooting, including the assertion that she had not intentionally fired the gun. These details were supported by the testimony of a firearms expert. Ms. Rock's testimony, however, was excluded because Arkansas had a per se rule excluding the admission of a criminal defendant's hypnotically refreshed testimony. On appeal, the U.S. Supreme Court held that an absolute prohibition of hypnotically refreshed testimony violates Fifth, Sixth, and Fourteenth Amendment rights. Specifically, it violates the right to be heard, the right to confront witnesses, and the right to testify on one's own behalf. The

Court ruled that admissibility of such testimony should be admitted on a case-by-case basis and cannot be barred by a blanket rule.

DAUBERT V. MERRELL DOW PHARMACEUTICALS, 509 U.S. 579 (1993)

Link to case: http://caselaw.lp.findlaw.com/scripts/getcase.pl?navby=case&court=us&vol=509&page=579

Question: Is *Frye v. U.S.* the appropriate standard for admitting scientific evidence into a federal court?

Answer: No.

Jason Daubert and Eric Schuller, minor children, and their parents sued Merrell Dow Pharmaceuticals for serious birth defects they alleged were caused by the mothers' taking of the antinausea medication Bendectin. Dow's expert opined that, based on all published studies, the drug was not teratogenic in humans. Daubert and others presented eight experts who, based on "reanalysis" of studies, opined that the drug could be teratogenic. Both the district court and the U.S. Court of Appeals for the Ninth Circuit found that the eight experts' testimonies did not meet the *Frye* test. On appeal, the U.S. Supreme Court unanimously found that the *Frye* test had been superseded by the Federal Rules of Evidence (first enacted in 1975), although a minority expressed disagreement as to how prescriptive the Court should be with regard to criteria for judicial gatekeeping. The majority of justices, however, agreed that the new rules require the trial judge to determine, through an assessment of an expert's evidence, that expert testimony "rests on a reliable foundation" and is "relevant" to understanding or determining an issue at hand. The Court offered a list of guidelines for admissibility of scientific testimony that focus on the methods, rather than the conclusions, of an expert's evidence. These guidelines are as follows: (1) Are the methods and/or rationale scientifically valid? (2) Has the theory been subject to peer review or publication? (3) Can or has the theory been tested? (4) What is the theory's or technique's known or potential error rate? (5) Are there standards that relate to the technique? (6) Is there widespread acceptance of the technique in the scientific community?

GENERAL ELECTRIC V. JOINER, 522 U.S. 136 (1997)

Link to case: http://caselaw.lp.findlaw.com/scripts/getcase.pl?navby=case&court=us&vol=522&page=136

Question: Should an appellate court use the "abuse of discretion" standard in reviewing a trial court's decision to admit or exclude expert testimony?

Answer: Yes.

Robert Joiner claimed that his work exposed him to hazardous polychlorinated biphenyl (PCBs) and their derivatives and that such exposure "promoted" his developing lung cancer. The District Court in Georgia granted summary judgment for General Electric based in part on the failure of Mr. Joiner's experts to show a link between PCBs and small-cell lung cancer. The judge found that the referenced animal and human studies either were not sufficiently relevant to Mr. Joiner's circumstances or were misinterpreted by Mr. Joiner's experts to bolster his claims. The court found that the expert opinion was speculative and *ipse dixit* (just because the expert said it was true). The U.S. Court of Appeals for the Eleventh Circuit reversed this decision, finding that the district court had overstepped its role by ruling on conclusions of experts rather than the "legal reliability" of evidence. The U.S. Supreme Court then reversed the court of appeals, unanimously agreeing that "abuse of discretion" (a judge's failure to properly consider a fact or law) is the appropriate standard for appellate review and that the district court had properly considered these issues.

KUMHO TIRE CO. V. CARMICHAEL, 526 U.S. 137 (1999)

Link to case: http://scholar.google.com/scholar_case?
case=11404623739922196630

Question: Does the *Daubert* decision apply to testimony from engineers and nonscientific testimony?

Answer: Yes.

Patrick Carmichael claimed that the minivan he was driving had a defective tire, made by Kumho Tire Co., that blew out and caused a motor vehicle accident that led to the death of one of the passengers and severe injury to others. He relied heavily on the expert opinion of a tire failure analyst, Dennis Carlson, Jr. The district court found initially and again on review that key technical evidence was not admissible under *Daubert* because it did not meet the reliability standards (e.g., scientifically reliable methodology, subject to peer review, known error rate) established in that case. The U.S. Court of Appeals for the Eleventh Circuit reversed the decision and remanded it for further consideration, stating that the district court should not have applied a "*Daubert* analysis" to a case that did not involve scientific evidence. The U.S. Supreme Court subsequently reversed the appellate decision and put to rest any doubt that *Daubert* applied to all expert testimony, including that which is not explicitly "scientific." Inasmuch as the Federal Rules of Evidence explicitly reference "scientific, technical and other specialized knowledge," all expert evidence is subject to judicial gatekeeping. The Court wrote that trial judges might apply the factors recommended by *Daubert* for reviewing scientific evidence to nonscientific evidence.

BUCK V. DAVIS, 137 S. CT. 759, 197 L. ED. 2D 1 (2017)

Link to case: https://www.supremecourt.gov/opinions/16pdf/15-8049_f2ah.pdf

Question: Can a finder of fact consider the race of a defendant in determining his future dangerousness for the purposes of sentencing, if a testifying expert considers it relevant?

Answer: No.

Duane Buck was convicted of capital murder in Texas for killing his former girlfriend and her friend. In capital cases, Texas law requires that the jury unanimously find, beyond a reasonable doubt, a probability that the defendant would commit future criminal acts of violence that would constitute a continuing threat to society. Buck's court-appointed lawyers called two psychologists to testify as experts to refute evidence of Buck's criminal history, lack of remorse, and alleged domestic abuse. Both concluded that Buck was unlikely to commit further violent acts, but one suggested that the fact Buck is black was relevant to the "future dangerousness" question. That expert stated that he considered demographic factors, including race, in his analysis and that, statistically, minorities are overrepresented in the criminal justice system. On cross-examination, the prosecution clarified that the expert's opinion was that the race factor "black" increased the likelihood of future dangerousness. After being sentenced to death by a jury and a denial of postconviction relief in state court, Buck filed for relief in federal court and asserted that the introduction of the racially biased testimony violated his right to effective counsel.

The U.S. Supreme Court granted certiorari and reversed and remanded Buck's case, finding that he had made a sufficient showing of ineffective assistance of counsel. The majority found that the testimony unambiguously appealed to a pernicious racial stereotype and would have likely had a powerful influence on jurors. The fact that the defense introduced the testimony gave it even further prejudicial weight as an admission against interest. The Court noted that there was a reasonable probability that Buck was sentenced to death in part based on his race and held that the district court's denial of Buck's motion for habeas relief was an abuse of discretion. To punish someone based on an immutable characteristic, the Court noted, "is a disturbing departure from a basic premise of our criminal justice system: Our law punishes people for what they do, not who they are."

CHAPTER 5

Questions on Mental Health Practice Guidelines

QUESTIONS

1. In order to pass the "*Frye* test," experts must be able to:
    A. Show that their peers have accepted the science used in testimony
    B. Present scientific evidence to the court in support of their testimony
    C. Demonstrate their scientific tests in court
    D. Present published papers or books that support their opinion
    E. Present their own publications supporting their opinions

2. In multiple appellate court decisions, the broadest guiding principal defining a psychiatrist's duty to protect a third party from a dangerous patient has been formulated as follows:
    A. Only when the name of a specific potential victim is identified does a psychiatrist incur a duty to protect.
    B. Only when a specific potential victim is identified does a psychiatrist incur a duty to protect.
    C. Only when a specific threat is made in the presence of the psychiatrist is a duty incurred.
    D. A psychiatrist has a duty to protect any class of persons who may be foreseeably harmed by a dangerous patient.

3. Hypnotically refreshed testimony may have usefulness:
    A. In guaranteeing the truth of repressed memory
    B. In accurately relaying very specific forgotten details
    C. In helping a subject relax and concentrate in order to better relay information
    D. In avoiding coerced testimony

4. "Abuse of discretion" in the context of the law means:
   A. A judge inappropriately applies the law.
   B. A judge abuses his or her discretion in evaluating evidence for admission.
   C. A judge decides arbitrarily or blatantly in error about evidentiary admissibility.
   D. All of the above.

5. It is more difficult to obtain adequate informed consent for experiments with involuntarily committed patients because:
   A. A high risk-to-benefit ratio requires greater understanding.
   B. Involuntarily committed patients may not be as informed.
   C. A lack of liberty requires procedural protections regarding informed consent.
   D. Involuntarily committed patients may have less monitoring.
   E. Involuntarily confined patients live in an "inherently coercive" environment, which might make it difficult for them to voluntarily consent.

6. The *Daubert* majority recommended that the judge conducting a preliminary *Daubert* hearing inquire about:
   A. Whether the science has been tested
   B. Whether the science has been peer reviewed and published
   C. Whether the science has a known or potential rate of error
   D. Whether the science has been generally accepted
   E. All of the above

7. When a psychiatrist believes that his or her patient/client poses an imminent threat to a third party, the duty to warn that third party:
   A. Has been established at a federal level by a U.S. Supreme Court decision
   B. Has been established as a federal law by act of Congress
   C. Has developed from state-specific case law that is binding only at a state level
   D. Was first outlined and advocated by the American Psychiatric Association

8. Hypnotically refreshed testimony:
   A. Is equivalent in reliability to a test for blood type
   B. Has well-established validity
   C. Is treated the same in virtually all jurisdictions
   D. Is available only in cases involving homicide crimes
   E. Has the potential to be unreliable

9. Under *Frye*, a psychiatric expert's testimony that contradicted a statement in the *Diagnostic and Statistical Manual of Mental Disorders* (DSM) would be most problematic if that expert had testified that the *DSM* is:
   A. Instructive
   B. Commonly used
   C. Written by experts in the field
   D. Authoritative
   E. Merely a guide in formulating a diagnosis

10. You have been treating a woman in your private practice for the past 5 years. She is a 69-year-old retired widow who lives with her son. During your session, you notice that she has a black eye covered with makeup and bruises on her arms. During therapy, she breaks down crying and divulges that her son has been beating her up. She begs you not to say anything to the authorities because she feels that she is financially dependent on her son and scared to live alone. What is the most appropriate way to handle this confidentiality situation?
   A. Reassure her that you will maintain confidentiality and provide her with a pamphlet of community support resources for battered women.
   B. Validate her fears and reassure her that Health Insurance Portability and Accountability Act of 1996 (HIPAA) laws prohibit you from sharing any unauthorized clinical information.
   C. Invite the son to her next therapy appointment to work through conflicts that may be occurring in the home.
   D. Validate her fears but inform her that this is a case of elder abuse and you need to report this abuse to the authorities for her safety.
   E. Inform her that as a psychiatrist, you are required to maintain her confidentiality. However, you will inform her internist, who may decide to report the abuse to the authorities.

11. As a result of the *Daubert, Joiner,* and *Kumho Tire* decisions, Rule 702 of the Federal Rules of Evidence has been amended to include which condition for admissibility of expert testimony?
   A. The expert's knowledge is limited to information based only on academic work and not on experience.
   B. Testimony is based on precedent from relevant case law.
   C. Testimony is the product of reliable principles and methods.
   D. The expert received training at a reputable medical school.

12. Physician/patient privilege belongs to:
   A. The patient's defense attorney
   B. The prosecuting attorney
   C. The patient's treating clinician
   D. The patient
   E. The patient's next of kin

13. Modern informed consent standards regarding medical decisions are primarily driven by the concept of:
    A. Autonomy
    B. Paternalism
    C. Justice
    D. Beneficence
    E. Competence

14. A mental health expert's concerns about the future of mental health testimony under the *Daubert* standard might include:
    A. Likelihood of "junk" science being admitted into evidence
    B. Role of the judge as gatekeeper
    C. A judge's reticence to admit a complicated but generally accepted psychological test
    D. All of the above

15. In federal courts, hypnotically refreshed testimony offered by defendants is:
    A. Inadmissible absent a showing of undue hardship
    B. Admissible subject to the Federal Rules of Evidence
    C. Admissible under the *Frye* standard
    D. Inadmissible under the *Daubert* standard

16. In, the Delaware Supreme Court agreed that Dr. Naidu's decision to discharge a psychiatric patient was the proximate cause of Mr. Laird's death because:
    A. The patient was discharged the same day his psychotic behavior led to Mr. Laird's death.
    B. The patient was discharged only a month before his psychotic behavior led to Mr. Laird's death.
    C. The court found that temporal span alone was not a sole determination of proximate cause.
    D. None of the above.

17. A man with chronic schizophrenia is evaluated in the emergency room and appears to be actively hallucinating. He says that he wants to sign himself into the hospital because the aliens tell him to do so. As a psychiatrist, you should:
    A. Allow the patient to voluntarily sign himself into the hospital.
    B. Sign the patient into the hospital as an involuntary patient.
    C. Assess for competence to sign voluntary admission forms and allow him to sign if competent.
    D. If not competent to sign voluntary papers, sign the patient into the hospital as an involuntary patient based only on his lack of competence.

18. As outlined in *Tarasoff*, the duty of a psychiatrist to protect a third party from a potentially dangerous patient:
    A. Is based on a psychotherapist's responsibility for his or her patient's actions as part of the legal treatment framework
    B. Arises from abilities psychiatrists are supposed to have to predict violence in the mentally ill
    C. Arises purely from a functional policy directive intended to minimize violent behavior in the mentally ill
    D. Is rooted in the special relationship between a psychotherapist and a patient, with an emphasis on foreseeability

19. Which of the following was a safeguard to ensure reliability of hypnotically refreshed testimony as established in *State v. Hurd*?
    A. Sessions should be conducted by a licensed psychiatrist or psychologist.
    B. The hypnotist should be independent of the parties involved.
    C. Sessions should be videotaped.
    D. Only the hypnotist and the subject should present during the session.
    E. All of the above.

20. Which of the following best describes the rules regarding child abuse reporting described in *State v. Andring*?
    A. Physician–patient privilege does not extend to group therapy because patients waive their confidentiality rights when they agree to participate in a group therapy format, which by nature requires open disclosure.
    B. Physician–patient privilege supersedes mandated reporting of child abuse if the perpetrator is engaged in mental health treatment.
    C. Mandated reporting of child abuse rarely preempts physician–patient privilege.
    D. The Federal Comprehensive Alcohol Abuse and Alcoholism Prevention, Treatment and Rehabilitation Act Amendments of 1974 included provisions to protect a patient's identity, diagnosis, prognosis, and treatment and preempts the state's mandated reporting requirements.
    E. Federal laws designed to protect the identity, diagnosis, prognosis, and treatment of patients engaged in alcohol or drug treatment are preempted by state-mandated reporting of child abuse requirements.

21. Informed consent must be:
    A. Voluntary
    B. Informed
    C. Competent
    D. All of the above

22. Which of the following is true regarding mandated reporting requirements?
    A. They include requirements to provide referrals and treatment to appropriate aftercare services.
    B. Physicians and psychologists are required to provide informed consent on evidence-based, trauma-focused cognitive behavioral therapy.
    C. They are jurisdiction dependent.
    D. They represent a discretionary duty for professionals.

23. Informed consent is required in which of the following situations?
    A. Before prescribing standing antipsychotic medications
    B. Before seclusion in the hospital
    C. Before administering an emergency intramuscular injection for dangerousness
    D. When the patient is admitted to a hospital involuntarily

24. The *Kumho Tire* opinion suggests that expert testimony based on clinical experience would be:
    A. Inadmissible on its face
    B. More highly scrutinized than scientific or technical expert testimony
    C. Admissible only when there is proof that it is scientific
    D. Subject to the same inquiry to assure reliability and relevance as other testimony
    E. Exempt from *Daubert*

25. Various state appellate courts have found which of the following as evidence of negligence in failing to exercise reasonable care to discharge the duty to protect third persons from a potentially dangerous patient?
    A. Failing to adequately review records related to a patient's past psychiatric history prior to discharging the patient
    B. Failing to consider involuntarily hospitalizing a voluntary patient and agreeing to discharge him instead without a reasonable aftercare plan
    C. Failing to address a patient's likelihood of relapsing on drugs of abuse and not taking prescribed medication after discharge
    D. All of the above

26. The following statement best reflects the reasoning for the ruling in *State v. Andring*:
    A. A patient's self-incriminating statements made during group therapy are different than those made during individual therapy and are therefore admissible to a court of law.
    B. The standard of confidentiality that protects physician–patient privilege during testimony in a trial is different than the standard for cooperating with law enforcement during an investigation of sexual abuse.
    C. Mental health treatment records are not considered to be protected by physician–patient privilege.
    D. Group therapy treatment records are protected by physician–patient confidentiality.
    E. When alleged perpetrators are enrolled in sexual offender treatment, they waive their right to confidentiality.

27. What is the significance of the following statement from the majority's decision in *Tarasoff*: "The protective privilege ends where the public peril begins"?
    A. A psychiatrist's duty to protect others from a dangerous patient is ultimately limited by public policy arguments protecting the confidential nature of the doctor–patient relationship.
    B. A psychiatrist's duty to protect the confidential nature of communications with a patient is ultimately limited by the need to protect the public from a potential and foreseeable danger.
    C. A psychiatrist's responsibility to the public is ultimately greater than his responsibility to keep one particular patient safe.
    D. A psychiatrist must protect his privilege to practice his profession but must also keep the public safe from psychiatric overclaim.

28. In which situation would a physician not have to give information regarding the risk of refusing a procedure?
    A. If the patient is a physician
    B. If the risk is commonly known
    C. If the risk is very rare
    D. If the patient is signing him- or herself in voluntarily to a hospital

ANSWERS

1. **A**

   The lower court denied *Frye*'s expert an opportunity to demonstrate the systolic blood pressure deception test in court, a denial affirmed by the appellate court. The court ruled that general acceptance of experts would determine whether this deception test could be accepted as scientifically sound. While presenting evidence from one's own research or that of peers might be useful, it is the general acceptance by the scientific community of one's opinions that is essential.

2. **D**

   Although state courts have varied in their definition of foreseeable victims, courts have found that psychiatrists are liable for failing to protect foreseeable victims when the name of the victim was not known (*Tarasoff v. Regents*), when no specific victim was threatened (*Naidu v. Laird* and *Lipari v. Sears*), and when no specific threat was made to the psychiatrist (*Jablonski v. U.S.*). The broadest formulation of a psychiatrist's duty to protect is that he or she take reasonable care to protect all foreseeable victims from a patient clinically judged to represent a danger to others.

3. **C**

   Despite the potential for hypnotically refreshed testimony to be unreliable, it has established usefulness in helping witnesses become more relaxed and to concentrate. Hypnosis does have the potential for coercion, and hypnotically refreshed testimony does not guarantee truth or the accuracy of details.

4. **D**

   "Abuse of discretion" is a term of art that refers to judicial inappropriateness in considering a law or a fact. Judges are given discretion in making all sorts of decisions, including the admissibility of evidence. "Abuse of discretion" is a standard of review used by appellate courts to review decisions of lower courts. The appellate court will typically find that the decision was an abuse of discretion if the discretionary decision was made in plain error.

5. **E**

   In *Kaimowitz v. Department of Mental Health for the State of Michigan*, the court ruled that involuntarily confined patients were unable to give consent for experimental psychosurgery. The court reasoned that a lack of liberty as related to involuntary commitment created an inherently coercive environment that made it more difficult to obtain adequate voluntary informed consent (E). A lack of liberty requiring greater procedural protections in informed consent is a general concept (C) but is not as specific an answer in describing why it is difficult to obtain informed consent for experimental research on involuntarily committed patients. A high risk-to-benefit ratio would require a greater level of understanding for informed consent but is not unique to involuntarily committed patients (A). Involuntarily committed patients could be as informed (B) and have equal monitoring (D) as other patients, and this does not explain the core difficulty of obtaining adequate informed consent for this group.

6. **E**

The Court gave some guidance regarding what the trial judge at a preliminary hearing might use to assess admissibility of evidence. The Court relied on scientific publications in suggesting these considerations. In the majority opinion, the *Frye* "standard" is one among several possible considerations, although evidence not generally accepted "may properly be viewed with skepticism."

7. **C**

In *Tarasoff v. Regents* (*Tarasoff v. Regents of University of California*, 17 Cal.3d 425, 31 Cal.Rptr. 14, 551 P.2d 334; 1976), the Supreme Court of California established the legal duty of psychotherapists to warn third parties when they believe their client poses an imminent threat.

Multiple subsequent appellate courts in various states have since found similarly in state-specific cases, but there is no U.S. Supreme Court precedent or national statute instituting a duty to protect on a federal level. The American Psychiatric Association filed an amicus brief arguing against imposing such a duty on psychotherapists in *Tarasoff*.

8. **E**

While hypnotically refreshed testimony is admissible, it does not have the same reliability status as a blood test. There is controversy around its use and validity, but courts have the option to adopt safeguards and guidelines as was done in *State v. Hurd* to ensure reliability as applied in a particular case. These guidelines do not have to be identical for all states. Although the two cases described, *Rock v. Arkansas* and *State v. Hurd*, involved homicide, hypnotically refreshed testimony is not limited to cases involving homicide.

9. **D**

Because the *Frye* test is the "general acceptance" test, the more generally accepted a piece of evidence, the less reliable any expert testimony that contradicts that piece of evidence would be. Once the expert has stated that a given text is authoritative, any evidence to the contrary would be less likely to pass muster under the *Frye* standard. Other descriptors that emphasize the limits of the *DSM* on a given issue (and, of course, other "generally accepted" evidence) would be more conducive to gaining the admissibility of an expert's statements that contradict the *DSM*.

10. **D**

In this case, you have an obligation to address the woman's abusive situation. The laws about reporting elder abuse (and child abuse) allow you to break confidentiality and report suspected abuse. Simply giving the patient a pamphlet is an insufficient intervention to protect her. HIPAA laws do not prohibit a clinician from reporting elder abuse. Inviting her son to her therapy session to address his abusive behavior would not be an appropriate intervention and would be insufficient to protect this patient. Passing this information on to her internist without reporting would not fulfill the required duty.

11. **C**

The Federal Rules of Evidence were amended in 2000 and again in 2011 to incorporate the *Daubert* decision. These amendments indicate the permanence in the shift toward judicial gatekeeping and scrutiny of expert testimony. Of the available choices, only C is correct. Expert knowledge can be based on relevant experience, case law is not considered a legitimate source of reliability for scientific evidence, and expert testimony does not have to be delivered by a medical doctor, much less one who trained at a reputable medical school.

12. **D**

Privilege is the patient's right to bar the clinician from testifying about information gathered in the course of treatment in legal settings (including trials, depositions, hearings, etc.). A useful mnemonic is "P = Privilege = Patient."

13. **A**

Paternalism relates to a right of the government to make policies to limit an individual's rights or liberties for the individual's own good. Paternalism is at odds with autonomy that relates to an individual's right to self-determination. From *Natanson v. Kline* to *Canterbury v. Spence* to *Truman v. Thomas*, informed consent decisions have moved away from paternalism (B) toward autonomy (A) as the driving concept. Justice is the fair treatment of individuals in a society (C). Beneficence is to do well to others (D). Neither is the driving concept behind informed consent decisions. An individual has to be competent (E) to give informed consent, but competence has not been used as an argument for informed consent.

14. **D**

These concerns (and more) have been extensively discussed in forums and publications since the *Daubert* decision. Fears about an inevitable "*Daubert* challenge" are common, and many papers address the potential or actual *Daubert* challenges and results when psychiatric issues, particularly novel concepts or tests, are at issue. *Daubert* can present the mental health expert with obstacles, but it can also provide an opportunity for the expert to define and clarify the scientific basis of his or her testimony.

15. **B**

Although the *Rock v. Arkansas* decision involved a state court issue, its holding involved the constitutional right of a defendant to testify on his own behalf and was decided by the U.S. Supreme Court; it is therefore applicable in federal courts. Thus, the Federal Rules of Evidence will govern the admissibility of any offered hypnotically refreshed testimony by a defendant. The *Daubert* criteria were incorporated into the Federal Rules of Evidence and do not automatically make hypnotically refreshed testimony inadmissible. Although the *Frye* opinion was a decision about expert testimony, it is no longer applicable in federal courts following the *Daubert* decision. "Undue hardship" is not a standard for hypnotically refreshed testimony admissibility.

16. **C**

More than 5 months after Mr. Putney was discharged from the Delaware State Hospital and while he was still psychotic, he intentionally drove his car into Mr. Laird's car, killing Mr. Laird. The trial court found Mr. Putney's negligent discharge as the proximate cause of Mr. Laird's death. The Delaware Supreme Court agreed, refuting the argument that too much time had elapsed to link the psychiatric discharge to the cause of death. As the court noted, "temporal span" by itself was insufficient to define proximate causation.

17. **C**

In *Zinermon v. Burch*, the U.S. Supreme Court decided that it was foreseeable that a person requesting treatment for mental illness may not be competent to give informed consent for voluntary hospitalization, which should be specifically assessed at the time of admission. As such, patients should not be automatically able to voluntarily sign themselves into a hospital without a competence evaluation (A).

Involuntary commitment criteria involve dangerousness *and* incompetence, not solely incompetence. A patient may not meet involuntary criteria (B), even if found incompetent to sign voluntary papers (D). In the situation posed in the question, the correct procedure would be (C), where the patient should be evaluated for competence to sign voluntary admission forms and, if competent, be allowed to sign. The psychiatrist should be aware of how competence to sign voluntary admission forms is defined by the controlling state statue and/or relevant case law. Psychosis, alone, may not render a person incompetent to sign.

18. **D**

The court in *Tarasoff* and other appellate courts have rooted the duty of a psychiatrist to protect a third party from a potentially dangerous patient in the special relationship between a psychotherapist and patient. This relationship puts a psychiatrist in a unique place to potentially foresee a danger to a particular third party or class of people, and in turn creates a duty to protect them. This duty is akin to that which a medical doctor has to the public when treating a potentially contagious patient. While the courts have acknowledged this duty, they have also voiced skepticism about psychiatry's actual ability to predict violence based on any scientific model. The duty arises in relation to specific foreseeable dangers; psychiatrists are otherwise not legally responsible for all of the conduct of their patients.

19. **E**

All of the choices presented in this question are safeguards that were presented in the *State v. Hurd* decision to help ensure reliability of hypnotically refreshed testimony. They were (1) sessions should be conducted by a licensed psychiatrist or psychologist; (2) parties involved should be independent; (3) information obtained by law enforcement should be written; (4) facts should be obtained from the subject before hypnosis; (5) sessions should be videotaped; and (6) only the hypnotist and subject should be present during the session.

20. **E**

Federal laws designed to protect the identity, diagnosis, prognosis, and treatment of patients engaged in alcohol or drug treatment are preempted by state-mandated reporting of child abuse requirements. While the Federal Comprehensive Alcohol Abuse and Alcoholism Prevention, Treatment and Rehabilitation Act Amendments of 1974 included provisions to protect a patient's identity, diagnosis, prognosis, and treatment, the court ruled that this act did not preempt child abuse reporting requirements. The perpetrator's engagement in mental health treatment is not relevant to reporting reasonable suspicions of abuse. It is false to state that mandated reporting of child abuse rarely preempts physician–patient privilege; this type of reporting is an explicit exception to that privilege. The court's holding was, in fact, that physician–patient privilege does extend to group therapy and was not preempted by the prosecution's evidentiary request for information in criminal proceedings.

21. **D**

Informed consent must involve each of the listed concepts (E). Informed consent must be voluntary (A) and free from coercion and duress. Problems with voluntariness arose in *Kaimowitz v. Department of Mental Health for the State of Michigan* where involuntarily committed patients were thought to be susceptible to coercion as related to their loss of liberty as involuntary patients. Informed consent must be informed (B), the amount of information having developed through case law in *Natanson v. Kline, Canterbury v. Spence*, and *Truman v. Thomas*. Finally, informed consent must be competent, and consent obtained when a patient is not competent may not be valid (C).

22. **C**

Mandated reporting requirements are jurisdiction dependent. They do not relate to duty to protect, and they do not require the mandated reporter to provide treatment referrals or aftercare services.

23. **A**

Clites v. Iowa found that informed consent was required prior to administration of antipsychotic medication. *Zinermon v. Burch* found that informed consent was required to sign voluntary paperwork, which should be assessed at the time of hospital admission; however, involuntary hospital commitment typically implies a lack of capacity and therefore does not required informed consent. Seclusion and emergency intramuscular injections are considered emergency situations for a patient who is an acute danger to self and others and would be considered exceptions to the informed consent requirement as described in *Canterbury v. Spence*.

24. **D**

According to the decision in *Daubert*, the role of judge as gatekeeper exists "to make certain that an expert, whether basing testimony upon professional studies or personal experience, employs in the courtroom the same level of intellectual rigor that characterizes the practice of an expert in the relevant field." *Daubert* factors can be applied to expert testimony, including psychiatric testimony, based on clinical experience and study. The U.S. Supreme Court in *Kumho Tire* stated that "a trial court should consider the specific factors identified in *Daubert* where there are reasonable measures of reliability of expert testimony."

25. **D**

All of the choices have been found as evidence of negligence to discharge a duty to protect (*Jablonski v. U.S.*, *Naidu v. Laird*, and *Petersen v. Washington*). Rather than proscribe a specific set of universal actions necessary to discharge this duty, courts have consistently found that a psychiatrist need only follow a standard of care that a reasonable psychiatrist would pursue in a similar clinical situation to protect a potential third-party victim from a foreseeable danger.

26. **D**

In *State v. Andring*, the court recognized that group therapy was no different than other forms of mental health treatment and, accordingly, was subject to the same levels of physician–patient confidentiality. Mental health treatment and group therapy records are both protected by physician–patient privilege. Patients are entitled to physician–patient confidentiality regardless of the type of treatment in which they are engaged.

27. **B**

When courts first outlined the scope of a psychiatrist's duty to protect third parties from foreseeable harm, many advocates of psychiatric treatment, including the American Psychiatric Association, argued that compromising the confidential nature of the communication between a patient and a treating mental health clinician would jeopardize the very efficacy of treatment itself. However, various state appellate courts have consistently held that this privilege of confidential communication is not without limits and ultimately may be sacrificed when a foreseeable harm can be averted by breaking confidentiality.

28. **1B**

Truman v. Thomas found that it constituted malpractice for a physician to fail to inform his or her patient of the consequences of refusing a medical procedure. Exceptions to disclosure include if the patient already knows the risk, such as if it is commonly known (e.g., getting sleepy from cough medicine). A rare risk (C) is not necessarily considered an exception because the risk could be significant, such as death, and be part of what a reasonable person would want to know.

SECTION II

Institutional Treatment Guidelines

CHAPTER 6

⌒◡⌒

Civil Commitment

ELIZABETH FORD

LAKE V. CAMERON, 364 F.2D 657 (1966)

Link to case: http://scholar.google.com/scholar_case?
case=16374362071956566586

Question: Can a civilly committed patient be involuntarily held in a hospital
if there are safe, less restrictive treatment alternatives available?

Answer: No.

Catherine Lake, a 60-year-old woman, was found wandering the streets of
Washington, DC. She was picked up by two policemen and taken to DC
General Hospital. She filed for a writ of habeas corpus in the DC Circuit
Court and was transferred to St. Elizabeth's Hospital (where Dale Cameron
was the superintendent) to await her civil commitment hearing. Her petition was denied without a hearing. In the meantime, the District of
Columbia passed the Hospitalization of the Mentally Ill Act, allowing
individuals with mental illness who are dangerous to themselves or others
to be either hospitalized or treated in a manner that maintains their best
interests and protects public safety. At Ms. Lake's subsequent commitment hearing, the examining psychiatrists found her to be of "unsound
mind" and suffering from mild dementia. She appealed to the U.S. Court
of Appeals, DC Circuit, which ruled that inpatient hospitalization was not
necessarily the least restrictive alternative or the most appropriate for Ms.
Lake, and the court held that the state had the obligation to explore these
less restrictive alternatives when considering involuntary hospitalization
for a patient. The court opined about the balance that might be obtained

from protecting Ms. Lake's liberty interests by enlisting family or community services to keep her safe. It wrote, "Deprivations of liberty solely because of dangers to the ill persons themselves should not go beyond what is necessary for their protection."

BAXSTROM V. HEROLD, 383 U.S. 107 (1966)

Link to case: http://scholar.google.com/scholar_case?case=17820943305043602552

Question: Can an individual being released from prison be civilly committed without being afforded the right to a jury determination of such commitment?

Answer: No.

Johnnie Baxstrom had been incarcerated at a New York prison on an assault conviction for some months when he was certified as "insane." He was subsequently transferred to Dannemora State Hospital, operated by the New York Department of Correction. At the termination of his criminal sentence, two physicians and Dr. Herold certified at surrogate court that Mr. Baxstrom should be civilly committed and transferred to the custody of the New York Department of Mental Hygiene (DMH). However, DMH did not think that Mr. Baxstrom was appropriate for their care system, and he therefore remained at Dannemora for more than 4 years after the completion of his criminal sentence. Mr. Baxstrom filed a writ of habeas corpus that he should be transferred to a civil facility if he was actually insane. The writ was denied several times by a state court and again by the Court of Appeals for New York. The U.S. Supreme Court granted certiorari and found that Mr. Baxstrom had been denied equal protection under the Fourteenth Amendment because he had been denied the right to jury review of the finding that he was mentally ill as is afforded all others who are facing civil commitment. The court did not find persuasive the state's argument that individuals evaluated for civil commitment at the end of penal sentences are categorically different than all others.

LESSARD V. SCHMIDT, 349 F. SUPP. 1078 (1972)

Link to case: http://scholar.google.com/scholar_case?case=16374362071956566586

Question: Should individuals facing civil commitment proceedings be entitled to due process rights similar to those in criminal proceedings?

Answer: Yes.

Alberta Lessard was brought to a mental health center in Milwaukee by two police officers. An emergency detention form was filed in order to detain her in the hospital. Three days later, with evidence presented from the officers related only to the initial reason for detention, the judge ordered 10 additional days of detention. At a subsequent hearing, upon petition of the mental health center claiming that Ms. Lessard should be "permanently committed" as a result of her schizophrenia, the judge ordered additional detention time. Ms. Lessard was not informed of any of these hearings or decisions. She filed a class action lawsuit in district court on behalf of herself and all involuntarily committed adults arguing that Wisconsin's involuntary commitment statute violated her due process rights. The court ruled in favor of Ms. Lessard, reasoning that because involuntary hospitalization was a significant deprivation of liberty in civil commitment hearings, the state was required to prove mental illness and dangerousness beyond a reasonable doubt and to ensure that less restrictive alternatives are not available. It also ruled that due process required that patients be given timely notice of their rights and have the right to legal counsel.

O'CONNOR V. DONALDSON, 422 U.S. 563 (1975)

Link to case: http://scholar.google.com/scholar_case?case=16877644373401713395

Question: Can a mentally ill patient be involuntarily committed to a hospital if he or she is not dangerous?

Answer: No.

Kenneth Donaldson had schizophrenia and was committed by his father under a relatively vague involuntary commitment statute to Florida State Hospital in Chattahoochee. While in the hospital for approximately 15 years, he was treated with "milieu therapy" but little else by way of therapy or medication. He did not behave in a manner that was dangerous to himself or others. Mr. Donaldson requested meetings with the superintendent of the hospital, Dr. J. B. O'Connor, as well as discharge, but was always denied. There were multiple people and organizations in the community willing to care for Mr. Donaldson. Dr. O'Connor eventually retired, Mr. Donaldson was released, and he filed suit, claiming that his constitutional right to liberty had been violated without providing required treatment. The district court and the U.S. Court of Appeals for the Fifth Circuit both found in favor of Mr. Donaldson and that he had a right to treatment as part of the Fourteenth Amendment. The U.S. Supreme Court heard the case but did not address the right to treatment issue. Instead, it found Mr. Donaldson's confinement unconstitutional because "a State cannot constitutionally confine without more a non-dangerous individual who is capable of surviving safely in freedom by himself or with the help of willing and responsible family members or friends."

ADDINGTON V. TEXAS, 441 U.S. 418 (1979)

Link to case: http://scholar.google.com/scholar_case?
case=1383560548954406906

Question: Is "clear and convincing evidence" the burden of proof for civil commitment?

Answer: Yes.

Frank Addington's mother filed a petition requesting the involuntary commitment of her son after he threatened her. He had a history of multiple prior hospitalizations. Mr. Addington requested a trial by jury to decide about his need for commitment. The judge instructed the jury to consider whether Mr. Addington was mentally ill and dangerous based on "clear and convincing evidence." At the 6-day trial, two psychiatrists who had evaluated Mr. Addington opined that he had schizophrenia and was "probably dangerous both to himself and to others." The jury found that he met criteria; he was indefinitely involuntarily committed to Austin State Hospital. Mr. Addington appealed to the Texas Court of Civil Appeals, claiming that due process required a finding "beyond a reasonable doubt" (criminal conviction). The Court of Civil Appeals agreed, but on further appeal, the Texas Supreme Court reversed and said that, in keeping with precedent, the burden of proof for civil commitment is "preponderance of the evidence." The U.S. Supreme Court granted certiorari, given the obvious confusion about this issue. In a unanimous decision, it found that an intermediate burden of proof by "clear and convincing evidence" was the most appropriate balance of individual rights and state's interests. A lower burden increased the risk of persons being confined for "mere idiosyncratic behavior," and beyond a reasonable doubt was burden that could not be met given the uncertainty of the science of psychiatry. The Court noted as well that "one who is suffering from a debilitating mental illness and in need of treatment is neither wholly at liberty nor free of stigma."

PARHAM V. J.R., 442 U.S. 584 (1979)

Link to case: http://caselaw.lp.findlaw.com/scripts/getcase.pl?navby=case& court=us&vol=442&page=584

Question: Is an adversarial hearing required for the hospitalization of a minor whose parents or guardian has requested such action?

Answer: No.

This case represented a class action in which J.R., a minor, was an appellee. He was removed from his parents' care at 3 months of age and was subsequently placed in seven successive foster homes. At age 7, J.R.'s seventh set of foster parents successfully applied for his admission to Central State Hospital in Georgia. Voluntary admission criteria per Georgia statute included the requirements of mental illness and suitability for hospital treatment, along with a requirement to discharge any child who has "sufficiently recovered" or improved such that hospitalization is no longer "desirable." Clinicians periodically reviewed J.R.'s need for hospitalization, and attempts were made to find placement for him in foster homes. He filed suit, along with others, requesting that he be transferred to a less restrictive setting. The district court agreed, finding that the mechanism for voluntary hospitalization of minors violated constitutional due process in light of the significant deprivation of liberty entailed in hospitalization. It found a "right after notice to be heard before an impartial tribunal" to be essential and that psychiatry was too "inexact" and sources of information potentially too unreliable to protect the liberty interests of children. It ordered that Georgia release at least 46 children into specialized community treatment. The U.S. Supreme Court heard the case and reversed the district court decision. It reasoned that in light of the medical questions raised in an application for voluntary admission, "due process is not violated by use of informal, traditional medical investigative techniques." It also noted the risks of intrusion into the parent–child relationship and the potential impact on the long-term treatment of the child with the introduction of an adversarial hearing. The Court also while inpatient hospitalization was potentially stigmatizing for a child, so too was remaining behaviorally unstable in the community. It did not find a compelling difference between requests for admission from natural parents of a child as compared with requests from state guardians (as in J.R.'s case).

CHAPTER 7

༄

Right to Die

ELIZABETH FORD

CRUZAN V. DIRECTOR OF MISSOURI DEPARTMENT OF MENTAL HEALTH, 497 U.S. 261 (1990)

Link to case: http://caselaw.lp.findlaw.com/scripts/getcase.pl?navby=case&court= us&vol=497&page=261

Question: Is it constitutionally acceptable for a state to require the burden of proof for removal of life-sustaining treatment from an incompetent individual to be clear and convincing evidence?

Answer: Yes.

Nancy Cruzan was in a motor vehicle accident in 1983 that resulted in severe anoxic brain injury and eventual decline into a persistent vegetative state that required artificial nutrition and hydration. Once it was clear that she would not recover, her parents asked the Missouri hospital where she was residing to terminate the artificial nutrition. Ms. Cruzan did not have any advance directives. By this time, Ms. Cruzan had been in a vegetative state for years. The hospital insisted on a court order for treatment termination; the state trial court granted that order, claiming a constitutional right to avoid "death-prolonging procedures" and in light of a prior conversation Ms. Cruzan had had with a friend about quality-of-life issues. Before the artificial feedings were discontinued, however, the Supreme Court of Missouri reversed the trial court based in part on findings that the evidence presented did not meet the "clear and convincing" standard required in Missouri and that Ms. Cruzan's parents could not automatically become her decision makers without required legal procedure. The U.S. Supreme

Court heard the case and found, in a 5–4 decision, that this standard was appropriate given the competing interests of Ms. Cruzan's liberty and the state's legitimate interest in preserving life. Following this decision, Ms. Cruzan's parents eventually produced further evidence of her wishes, and the Missouri court granted the removal of the feeding tube.

WASHINGTON V. GLUCKSBERG, 521 U.S. 702 (1997)

Link to case: http://scholar.google.com/scholar_case?case=17920279791882194984

Question: Does the ban on physician-assisted suicide of competent terminally ill adults in the State of Washington violate the Due Process Clause of the Fourteenth Amendment?

Answer: No.

Harold Glucksberg and three other physicians, along with three terminally ill patients and a nonprofit organization offering counseling to patients considering physician-assisted suicide, sued the State of Washington and claimed that Washington's ban on physician-assisted suicide was unconstitutional by violating Fourteenth Amendment liberty interests in making end-of-life decisions. The district court agreed and also found that the Washington law violated the Equal Protection Clause. A panel of judges from the U.S. Court of Appeals for the Ninth Circuit reversed and stated that there was no precedent for allowing someone to kill him or herself. The entire appellate court then reheard the case and changed its decision, finding that the Constitution allowed for a "right to die." The U.S. Supreme Court reversed the Ninth Circuit, reasoning that there is no tradition of a right to die in the United States; that Washington State has a legitimate interest in preserving life, protecting vulnerable patients, and preserving the medical profession; and that a right to die is not a fundamental liberty interest. The Court issued the opinions for this case and *Vacco v. Quill* on the same day, striking down both elements of the Fourteenth Amendment claims (substantive due process—*Washington*—and equal protection—*Vacco*).

VACCO V. QUILL, 521 U.S. 793 (1997)

Link to case: http://scholar.google.com/scholar_case?case=10644975876581235704

Question: Does an individual have a right to physician-assisted suicide under the Equal Protection Clause of the Fourteenth Amendment?

Answer: No.

Timothy Quill, Samuel Klagsbrun, and Howard Grossman were three physicians in New York who filed a suit, along with three terminally ill patients, against the state's attorney general, Dennis Vacco. The physicians reported that the New York State ban on physician-assisted suicide made it illegal for them to practice consistent with their standards by prescribing lethal doses of medication for their "mentally competent, terminally ill" patients. The physicians and patients argued an equal protection claim that competent patients were allowed to refuse life-sustaining treatment yet were not allowed to seek the assistance of a physician to end their life. The district court dismissed the case, finding a significant difference between intentional action to end life and a natural end to life. However, the U.S. Court of Appeals for the Second Circuit reversed and found Dr. Quill's and others' arguments compelling. The U.S. Supreme Court heard the case and in a unanimous decision found in favor of New York State. It wrote that mentally competent people were entitled to refuse life-sustaining treatment, but that "no one is permitted to assist a suicide." It did not find the two situations to be similar classes of individuals entitled to equal protection.

CHAPTER 8

Right to Treatment

BIPIN SUBEDI

ROUSE V. CAMERON, 373 F.2D 451 (1966)

Link to case: http://scholar.google.com/scholar_case?
case=10042825042511534924

Question: Do hospitalized insanity acquittees have a right to treatment?

Answer: Yes.

Charles Rouse was arrested in Washington, DC, carrying a 45-caliber re-
volver and 600 rounds of ammunition. He successfully pled insanity on
a misdemeanor weapons violation, a charge that carried a maximum
sentence of 1 year and was sent to St. Elizabeth's Hospital. While at St.
Elizabeth's, Mr. Rouse was only intermittently engaged in group/indi-
vidual therapy and was not prescribed medication. After 3 years of hospitalization, he petitioned Dale Cameron, the superintendent, for release on
the grounds that there was no basis for continued hospitalization if he was
not receiving treatment. The DC District Court denied a hearing, stating
that its jurisdiction was limited to determinations of sanity, not right to
treatment. The DC Court of Appeals agreed to hear the case and ruled that
a district code citing a statutory right to treatment for civilly committed
patients applied to insanity acquittees. In the ruling, Judge David Bazelon
stated that dangerousness determinations should be based on symptoms
of mental illness and not on the crime itself. He defined treatment broadly
as an "effort" to improve health and alluded to Rouse's right to treatment
under the Due Process Clause of the Fourteenth Amendment. The case was
reversed and remanded with instructions for the lower court to evaluate

the adequacy of the treatment being provided, as well as the continuing need for hospitalization.

WYATT V. STICKNEY, 344 F. SUPP. 373 (1972)

Link to case: http://scholar.google.com/scholar_case?
case=15111627758791375629

Question: Are individuals civilly committed for mental illness or mental retardation entitled, by the U.S. Constitution, to minimally adequate standards for psychiatric treatment?

Answer: Yes.

Ricky Wyatt, a patient at Bryce Hospital in Tuscaloosa, Alabama, sued the hospital over poor conditions and treatment on behalf of other patients confined at Bryce and several employees. At the time, Alabama ranked fiftieth in the United States in per-patient expenditures per day. In addition, state losses following a change in tobacco taxation led to the termination of 99 employees months prior to the initiation of the suit. The District Court in Alabama agreed that treatment was grossly deficient and gave the defendants 6 months to improve conditions; 6 months later, the court determined that the defendants had failed to do so. It ruled that confining an individual for therapeutic purposes while not providing adequate treatment was a violation of substantive due process under the Fourteenth Amendment. The court subsequently held formal hearings with mental health professionals to determine the minimal constitutional standards for the treatment of psychiatric inpatients. It determined that this included (1) a humane psychological and physical environment; (2) qualified staff in numbers sufficient to administer adequate treatment; and (3) individualized treatment plans. Requirements for staffing included two psychiatrists and 12 nurses per 250 patients. The same court extended this ruling to institutions caring for the mentally disabled shortly after.

YOUNGBERG V. ROMEO, 457 U.S. 307 (1982)

Link to case: http://scholar.google.com/scholar_case?
case=7713558129166322035

Question: Does the Fourteenth Amendment right to liberty include freedom from bodily restraint, safe conditions, and minimally adequate skills to reduce the need for restraint for intellectually disabled individuals who are civilly committed?

Answer: Yes.

Nicholas Romeo was a 33-year-old man with a mental capacity of an 18-month-old and an IQ score between 8 and 10. He had a history of violence and was committed to Pennhurst State School and Hospital in Pennsylvania after his father's death. At Pennhurst, Mr. Romeo suffered from multiple injuries on at least 63 occasions over 3 years. Mr. Romeo's mother filed suit against Mr. Youngberg, the superintendent at Pennhurst, claiming Eighth Amendment constitutional violations that Mr. Romeo was receiving inadequate care and had a right to safe conditions, freedom from bodily restraint, and minimally adequate skills development ("habilitation") to reduce the need for restraint. The jury found for Mr. Romeo, but the Court of Appeals for the Third Circuit reversed and remanded for a new trial, ruling that the Fourteenth Amendment's protection of liberty interests should be the guiding principle in the decision. The U.S. Supreme Court agreed to hear the case and ruled that institutionalized persons are dependent on the state and therefore have a significant liberty interest that implicates due process protections, including his right to treatment (habilitation) which herein was seen through the liberty lens, that is, diminishing the need for physical restraint. However, the Court also stated that "professional judgment"—an assessment of whether an action substantially deviated from the standard of care—was the appropriate measure of whether the state had met its duty.

CHAPTER 9

Right to Refuse Treatment

REBECCA LEWIS

APPLICATION OF THE PRESIDENT AND DIRECTORS OF GEORGETOWN UNIVERSITY, 331 F.2D 1000 (1964)

Link to case: http://law.justia.com/cases/federal/appellate-courts/F2/331/1010/445992/

Question: Does imminent danger of death trump an incompetent patient's religious objections to emergency medical treatment in the District of Columbia?

Answer: Yes.

Jesse Jones was a patient at Georgetown University Hospital in Washington, DC. Her husband brought her to the hospital for emergency care after she lost two-thirds of her blood from a ruptured ulcer. Blood transfusions were necessary to save her life, but Mrs. Jones and her husband refused to consent to the blood transfusions based on their religious beliefs as Jehovah's Witnesses. When death without transfusion became imminent, the hospital applied to the district court for permission to administer blood transfusions. The district court denied the application. The hospital then applied to Judge Wright as a member of the DC Circuit Court of Appeals for an emergency writ. Judge Wright confirmed the medical facts with the doctors. He spoke with Mrs. Jones's husband, who said that on religious grounds he would not approve a blood transfusion, but that if the court ordered the transfusion, the responsibility was not his. Judge Wright then tried to communicate with Mrs. Jones; her only audible reply was "against my will." Judge Wright found her incompetent to make medical decisions in her compromised state of health. He granted permission for blood transfusions "to save her life" and stated that death could have made the case moot.

SUPERINTENDENT OF BELCHERTOWN STATE SCHOOL ET AL. V. JOSEPH SAIKEWICZ, 370 N.E.2D 417 (1977)

Link to case: http://scholar.google.com/scholar_case?case=2165107287898894579

Question: Is substituted judgment an appropriate decision-making standard for a legally appointed guardian to employ when making medical decisions for his or her ward?

Answer: Yes.

Joseph Saikewicz, a resident of the Belchertown State School in Massachusetts, was 67 years old and had an IQ of 10. He was diagnosed with leukemia and was incapable of giving consent for treatment. The superintendent petitioned for appointment of a guardian ad litem to make treatment decisions. The guardian ad litem recommended that treatment for Mr. Saikewicz would not be in his best interests based on the following assessment: (1) the treatment (chemotherapy) would cause significant adverse effects that Mr. Saikewicz would not understand, (2) there was a low chance of remission, and (3) there would be only a limited extension of life if remission occurred. The probate court agreed with the substituted judgment of the guardian and ordered that no treatment be administered. Although Mr. Saikewicz died in the interim, the probate court requested review of this decision by the Supreme Court of Massachusetts. That court concluded that substituted judgment for incompetent patients was the appropriate decision-making standard and that "to presume that the incompetent person must always be subjected to what many rational and intelligent persons may decline is to downgrade the status of the incompetent person by placing a lesser value on his intrinsic human worth and vitality."

IN THE MATTER OF THE GUARDIANSHIP OF RICHARD ROE, III, 421 N.E.2D 40 (1981)

Link to case: http://masscases.com/cases/sjc/383/383mass415.html#back23

Question: Can a legally appointed guardian of a non-hospitalized individual in Massachusetts with mental illness consent to nonemergent administration of antipsychotic medication for that individual?

Answer: No.

Richard Roe III was diagnosed with paranoid schizophrenia as a teenager and was eventually hospitalized at Northampton State Hospital, where he refused antipsychotic medications. His father was appointed as guardian after his discharge from the hospital. The probate court ordered that Mr. Roe's father would have the authority to consent to forcible administration of medication. The guardian ad litem, appointed to represent Mr. Roe in the probate hearing, appealed. The Massachusetts Supreme Court held that the appointment of a guardian was warranted and that the evidence was appropriately tested under a "preponderance of the evidence" standard of proof. However, the court ruled that it was an error to empower the guardian (Mr. Roe's father) to consent for forcible administration of medications. The court concluded that, absent an emergency, in a noninstitutionalized patient, antipsychotic medications may be administered forcibly only when ordered by a judge using a substituted judgment standard. It determined that if the ward, if competent, would accept the medications, the judge should order administration. If determined that the substituted judgment would be to refuse treatment, then the judge should consider whether there is a state interest sufficient to override the decision to refuse (e.g., interest in preventing violence). If the judge finds that there is such a state interest, then an extended substituted judgment determination must be used to choose between options for satisfying this interest (e.g., involuntary commitment vs. forced medication).

RENNIE V. KLEIN, 720 F.2D 266 (3D CIR. 1983) (ON REMAND)

Link to case: http://scholar.google.com/scholar_case?
case=11241063757300199813

Question: In New Jersey, is a court order required for the non-emergency administration of antipsychotic medication for individuals civilly committed for psychiatric treatment?

Answer: No.

During his twelfth hospitalization at a New Jersey state hospital, John Rennie initiated a suit claiming a constitutional right of involuntarily hospitalized mentally ill patients to refuse antipsychotic medications. The district court agreed. The U.S. Court of Appeals for the Third Circuit found that the constitutional right to refuse treatment existed, but it found that the administrative procedures outlined in New Jersey's Administrative Bulletin (which required a hospital administrative review prior to forcible administration of medications) provided adequate protection and satisfied due process. The court added that the medication administered must be the least restrictive treatment available. This decision was then appealed to the U.S. Supreme Court. The Court instructed the Third Circuit to reconsider the case in view of the Supreme Court's finding in *Youngberg v. Romeo*, which adopted a standard of "professional judgment" instead of the "least restrictive means." The New Jersey procedures require that the physician explain reasons for medication, the benefits and risks of medication, and alternative courses of action. Additionally, the proposed treatment must be reviewed and approved by other professional staff. Upon reconsideration, the Third Circuit found that the New Jersey regulations satisfied the professional judgment standard. This case represents a treatment-driven approach to establishing a patient's right to refuse treatment.

ROGERS V. COMMISSIONER, 458 N.E.2D 308 (1983)

Link to case: http://freedom-center.org/pdf/rogersruling.pdf

Question: In Massachusetts, does treatment of an involuntarily committed patient who is refusing psychiatric medication require a court order?

Answer: Yes.

Rubie Rogers was one of the plaintiffs in a class action against the commissioner of the Department of Mental Health in Massachusetts that challenged the practice of medicating patients against their will. The district court found that forcibly medicating hospitalized patients in nonemergency situations was prohibited, but it denied damages. Both parties appealed. The U.S. Court of Appeals for the First Circuit affirmed the denial of damages and also affirmed that mentally ill patients have a constitutionally protected right to refuse treatment. However, the court of appeals expanded the meaning of emergency to allow for "physician discretion" in deciding whether there was a likelihood of physical harm and to consider if a patient's health would significantly deteriorate without medications. The U.S. Supreme Court granted certiorari, vacated the judgment, and remanded the case to the court of appeals to specify how the patient's rights were protected under existing Massachusetts law. The opinion in this case represents the response by the Supreme Judicial Court of Massachusetts to specific questions certified to it by the court of appeals. The Massachusetts court responded as follows: (1) competency and substituted judgment determinations must be made in court by a judge; (2) a substituted judgment treatment decision must be made before a hospitalized patient can be forcibly medicated; and (3) emergencies (e.g., preventing violence or preventing the immediate and irreversible deterioration of serious mental illness) are exceptions to these requirements. This case is an example of a rights-driven approach to a patient's right to refuse treatment (in contrast to *Rennie v. Klein*—a treatment-driven approach).

CHAPTER 10

Questions on Institutional Treatment Guidelines

QUESTIONS

1. What does the principle of "least restrictive alternative" refer to?
   A. Keeping someone in jail or prison no longer than his or her sentence
   B. Allowing individuals the freedom to choose their treatment setting
   C. The minimum restriction of liberty (e.g., force, coercion, or confinement) needed to ensure safety
   D. Using justice as a means of enforcing the law

2. In order to remove life-sustaining treatment from an incompetent individual without existing advance directives, the required burden of proof is:
   A. Preponderance of the evidence
   B. Clear and convincing evidence
   C. Beyond a reasonable doubt
   D. With reasonable medical certainty

3. What is substituted judgment?
   A. When a guardian or judge determines the choice a currently incompetent individual would make if he or she were competent
   B. When a doctor is asked to determine the most medically appropriate treatment for an incompetent individual
   C. When a judge is asked to determine what treatment choice the majority of people in the same medical position as the incompetent individual would make
   D. When an incompetent individual's next of kin makes the decision about treatment for that individual

4. What U.S. Supreme Court case made dangerousness a required part of the standard for civil commitment?
   A. *Lessard v. Schmidt*
   B. *Lake v. Cameron*
   C. *O'Connor v. Donaldson*
   D. *Addington v. Texas*

5. The final decision in *Youngberg v. Romeo* was rendered by which court?
   A. U.S. District Court
   B. U.S. Court of Appeals
   C. U.S. Supreme Court
   D. Family court

6. Is physician-assisted suicide allowable under the American Medical Association (AMA) guidelines?
   A. Yes.
   B. No.
   C. The AMA does not comment on physician-assisted suicide.
   D. The AMA allows physician-assisted suicide in certain circumstances.

7. In *Rouse v. Cameron*, the Washington, DC, statutory right to treatment that applied to civilly committed patients was found to also apply to which other class of individuals?
   A. Individuals with developmental disabilities
   B. Insanity acquittees
   C. Prisoners
   D. Pretrial detainees

8. As delineated in *Application of the President and Directors of Georgetown University*, can medical professionals provide emergency life-saving medical treatment to an incompetent person against his or her will?
   A. Yes. Physicians are always permitted to treat incompetent individuals, as long as it is the appropriate medical treatment, even in a nonemergency situation.
   B. Yes. If the medical treatment is life-saving and there is imminent risk of death, physicians can provide the treatment.
   C. Yes, but only if there is a judicial court order for treatment.
   D. No. Medical professionals are never permitted to treat individuals against their will, even if the individual is incompetent.

9. In *Wyatt v. Stickney*, the U.S. District Court ruled that the minimal constitutional requirements for the treatment of committed patients were:
   A. Humane psychological and physical environment, qualified staff in numbers sufficient to administer adequate treatment, right to legal representation

B. Humane psychological and physical environment, qualified staff in numbers sufficient to administer adequate treatment, and adequate funding

C. Qualified staff in numbers sufficient to administer adequate treatment, individualized treatment plans, and adequate funding

D. Humane psychological and physical environment, qualified staff in numbers sufficient to administer adequate treatment, and individualized treatment plans

10. The U.S. Supreme Court has found which of the following to be a compelling argument against physician-assisted suicide?
   A. The difference between letting a patient die and making a patient die
   B. Competent individuals should have a right to choose their manner of death
   C. Competent people can refuse life-saving treatments
   D. All of the above

11. The minimum legal burden of proof for civil commitment in the United States is:
   A. Beyond reasonable doubt
   B. Reasonable medical certainty
   C. Preponderance of the evidence
   D. Clear and convincing evidence
   E. Without due cause

12. *In the Matter of Richard Roe, III* was a case involving an outpatient minor. Based on that case, does a guardian have the authority to consent to forcible medication of his or her ward?
   A. No. Medications cannot be administered against someone's will if the person is not hospitalized.
   B. No. Only a court can determine if forcible medication can be ordered for an outpatient.
   C. Yes. The courts appoint a guardian, and this guardian then has the authority to consent for medically appropriate treatment, even if it is against the ward's wishes.
   D. Yes. A review between the guardian and the ward's physician is appropriate.

13. What type of circumstance allows an individual the right to an adversarial hearing?
   A. If a minor, when one's parents apply for voluntary admission
   B. All voluntary admissions, regardless of age of the individual
   C. When facing involuntary hospitalization
   D. When a request for release from a medical unit is denied

14. According to the U.S. Supreme Court, physician-assisted suicide:
    A. Is constitutional under the Fourteenth Amendment
    B. Reasonably allows an individual to exercise his or her autonomy
    C. Should not be an issue decided at the Supreme Court level
    D. Is not rationally related to legitimate government interests
    E. Is akin to allowing a patient to die of natural causes

15. Of the following choices, which legal or ethical principles are most at odds in civil commitment proceedings?
    A. Nonmaleficence versus police power
    B. Beneficence versus autonomy
    C. Autonomy versus police power
    D. Autonomy versus nonmaleficence
    E. Justice versus beneficence

16. According to *Washington v. Glucksberg* and *Vacco v. Quill*, state bans on physician-assisted suicide do not violate:
    A. The Eighth Amendment
    B. The First Amendment
    C. The Fourteenth Amendment
    D. The Sixth Amendment
    E. The Second Amendment

17. In *Rennie v. Klein*, a treatment-driven model of adjudicating cases involving treatment refusal was adequate. What reasoning was used?
    A. The courts should decide these cases based on substituted judgment.
    B. Professional judgment should guide treatment refusal decisions.
    C. The judicial system should tightly monitor all clinical decisions regarding treatment refusal.
    D. Specific treatment should be implemented once an order to medicate someone against his or her will is obtained.

18. Protections for patients involuntarily committed to a psychiatric hospital include:
    A. Right to legal representation
    B. Right to leave the hospital against medical advice
    C. Right to choose their doctor
    D. Right to choose the hospital to which they are committed

19. A hospitalized patient of yours is in a persistent vegetative state fol-
    lowing a major car accident and is receiving artificial nutrition and hy-
    dration to stay alive. He does not have any written advance directives,
    but his older brother wishes to remove the feeding tube and allow his
    brother's life to take a natural course, even if that ends in death. What
    would be the best first step?
    A. Tell the brother that the tube can never be removed.
    B. Consult the hospital risk management department.
    C. Talk to other family members about their wishes.
    D. Remove the feeding tube.

20. Does an incompetent individual have the right to refuse life-prolonging
    medical treatment?
    A. Yes, but only if that individual had made his or her desire to avoid
       such treatment known prior to becoming incompetent.
    B. Yes, but only if it is shown that the majority of people in a similar
       situation would refuse such treatment.
    C. No. If treatment can prolong life, and the individual is incompe-
       tent, he or she cannot refuse such treatment.
    D. Yes. Even if the individual has never been competent, a legally ap-
       pointed guardian can make the decision.

21. Which of the following statements best describes the procedure for
    civilly committing an individual being released from prison?
    A. The individual must be assessed by at least three psychiatrists, all
       board certified by the ABPN.
    B. The individual should be afforded the right to a jury trial the same
       as for nonprisoners being civilly committed.
    C. The individual should be released from prison into the community
       before being assessed for civil commitment.
    D. The individual should be found in need of civil commitment beyond
       a reasonable doubt.

22. The U.S. Supreme Court defined what standard for determining
    Fourteenth Amendment violations of due process for civilly com-
    mitted, intellectually disabled individuals?
    A. Substantial necessity
    B. Professional judgment
    C. Compelling necessity
    D. Reasonable medical certainty
    E. Preponderance of the evidence

ANSWERS

1. **C**

   "Least restrictive alternative" is a concept that describes respecting an individual's autonomy and therefore only infringing on that person's liberty as much as is necessary for safety. It is mentioned frequently in legal cases involving civil commitment and patient rights. Answer (D) relates to issues of therapeutic jurisprudence and police power, neither of which is directly related to least restrictive alternative.

2. **B**

   The issue was decided in the U.S. Supreme Court case *Cruzan v. Director of Missouri Department of Mental Health* in 1990. It involved a woman in a persistent vegetative state who did not have advance directives and whose parents wished to withdraw life-sustaining nutrition and hydration. The Court reasoned that the state had a strong interest in preserving life and that the "clear and convincing" standard appropriately weighted that interest against an individual's liberty interest. Answers (A) and (C) are lower and higher standards of proof, respectively. Answer (D) is the level of certainty physicians use in offering expert opinions.

3. **A**

   Substituted judgment is used to determine what an incompetent individual would choose if he or she were competent. In *In the Matter of the Guardianship of Richard Roe, III*, the Massachusetts Supreme Court outlined the important factors to consider when determining substituted judgment: (1) the ward's expressed preferences, (2) the ward's religious beliefs, (3) the impact upon the ward's family, (4) the probability of adverse side effects of treatment, (5) the consequences if treatment is refused, and (6) the prognosis with treatment.

4. **C**

   O'Connor v. Donaldson was a U.S. Supreme Court case that highlighted dangerousness, along with mental illness, as the required criteria for civil commitment. *Lessard v. Schmidt* (Wisconsin) and *Lake v. Cameron* (Washington, DC) were not U.S. Supreme Court cases. *Addington v. Texas* defined the burden of proof for involuntary psychiatric hospitalization but did not define the clinical requirements.

5. **C**

   The U.S. Supreme Court, in *Youngberg v. Romeo*, recognized that persons subject to involuntary commitment proceedings have a liberty interest, protected under the Due Process Clause, to safety and to freedom from bodily restraint. The court also found that Mr. Romeo had a constitutional right to minimally adequate habilitation (i.e., treatment).

The Alabama District Court ruled in *Wyatt v. Stickney*, and the DC Court of Appeals ruled in *Rouse v. Cameron*. Family courts do not have the jurisdiction to address constitutional matters.

6. **B**

The AMA comments on physician-assisted suicide in Opinion 2.211 (http://www.ama-assn.org//ama/pub/physician-resources/medical-ethics/code-medical-ethics/opinion2211.page). In it, the AMA finds that the practice is "incompatible with the physician's role as healer." It does not list any exceptions to this position.

7. **B**

Charles Rouse was an insanity acquittee who petitioned for release and stated that he was not receiving treatment where he had been hospitalized following his acquittal. Although a district court statute clearly outlined a right to treatment for civilly committed patients, it was unclear, prior to this case, if this applied to those who were found not criminally responsible secondary to mental illness. In *Rouse v. Cameron*, the DC Circuit Court of Appeals ruled that once found not responsible, Mr. Rouse's confinement was based on his mental illness and, therefore, he had the same right to treatment. The case does not discuss incarcerated individuals or individuals with developmental disabilities.

8. **B**

In *Application of the President and Directors of Georgetown University*, a patient was at imminent risk of death from a bleeding ulcer and was refusing blood transfusions. A judge determined that the patient was incompetent, and that treatment should be provided to save her life. He noted that waiting for a court hearing would have mooted the issue because the patient would die before a hearing. Physicians are not permitted to treat incompetent patients against their will in nonemergency settings. Instead, they must consult a legal surrogate (e.g., power of attorney, court-appointed guardian).

9. **D**

In *Wyatt v. Stickney*, the court ruled that patients had the rights outlined in (D) and provided specific guidelines in the appendix of the ruling. Lack of funding was not considered to be a valid excuse in failing to provide the necessary services.

10. **A**

In their decisions in *Washington v. Glucksberg* and *Vacco v. Quill*, the U.S. Supreme Court emphasized the difference between allowing a patient to die naturally (e.g., not initiating extraordinary measures) and causing a patient to die (physician-assisted suicide). Answers (B) and (C) are arguments in favor of physician-assisted suicide but were not compelling enough to the Court.

11. **D**

Since *Addington v. Texas*, the minimum burden of proof for the fact finder (e.g., judge or jury) in a civil commitment proceeding is "clear and convincing evidence." The U.S. Supreme Court considered the standard of "beyond reasonable doubt" (used in criminal matters) so high that it would limit access to hospitalization for mentally ill patients because few would reach that burden of proof. "Preponderance of the evidence" (more likely than not) was considered so low that the autonomy rights of individuals with mental illness would not be protected, and unfair hospitalizations would occur. "Clear and convincing evidence" was considered a reasonable compromise. "Reasonable medical certainty" is the standard that an evaluating clinician must use in determining whether or not to initiate civil commitment. It is equivalent to "more likely than not." "Without due cause" is not a recognized standard.

12. **B**

In *In the Matter of the Guardianship of Richard Roe, III*, the father of Richard Roe was appointed his guardian after his discharge from a state hospital and authorized to consent to forcible administration of antipsychotic medications for Richard Roe. This was appealed, and the Massachusetts Supreme Court found that in a noninstitutionalized patient, absent an emergency, antipsychotic medications could be administered forcibly only when ordered by a judge.

13. **C**

Individuals facing involuntary hospitalization have a right to an adversarial hearing, among other due process rights (see *Lessard v. Schmidt*). The case of *Parham v. J.R.* found that Georgia's practice of voluntary admission for minors was constitutional and did not require an adversarial hearing. Although *Parham* was a case about a class action related to minors, adults who request voluntary admission do not have a right to an adversarial hearing. Individuals who are admitted to a medical unit and are denied release upon request can, if competent and not in an emergency situation, sign out against medical advice without a hearing.

14. **D**

The U.S. Supreme Court heard two major state cases about physician-assisted suicide in 1997: *Washington v. Glucksberg* (Washington) and *Vacco v. Quill* (New York). In each, the Court found that the state could ban the procedure according to the Fourteenth Amendment. It was not swayed by arguments about an individual's right to die (autonomy). The Court found a significant difference between letting a patient die by natural causes and hastening his or her death (likened to killing a patient). Prominent arguments in each case were the respective state's reasonable and legitimate interests in preserving life and protecting vulnerable populations.

15. **C**

All of the ethical principles described are frequently considered in psychiatric practice; however, autonomy and police power are the most in conflict during civil commitment decisions. Autonomy means the ability to be one's own person and to act in one's own interests, regardless of the input from others. Police power is a right of the government to make policies that protect the safety and welfare of the community. In civil commitment decisions, a mentally ill individual's autonomy to make treatment decisions is balanced against the state's right to restrict the liberty of those who may be dangerous. Nonmaleficence is the concept in the Hippocratic Oath commonly known as "first, do no harm." It, along with beneficence (do what is in the best interests of the patient), is a common principle in clinical practice. Justice is the fair treatment of all individuals in a society.

16. **C**

Both cases were Fourteenth Amendment claims, but each emphasized a different part of the amendment. *Washington v. Glucksberg* was an equal protection claim, and *Vacco v. Quill* was a due process claim. The Eighth and Sixth Amendments are both related to criminal justice, the First Amendment has to do with freedom of speech and religion, and the Second Amendment has to do with a right to bear arms.

17. **B**

Rennie v. Klein exemplifies the treatment-driven model. In this case, it was found that a constitutional right to refuse treatment existed, but that the administrative procedures outlined in New Jersey's Administrative Bulletin (which required a hospital administrative review prior to forcible administration of medications) provided adequate protection of patients' rights and found that the decision to medicate a patient against his or her wishes must be the result of professional judgment (to protect the patient from inappropriate or unnecessary medication). *Rogers v. Commissioner* exemplifies the rights-driven model. In this case, the courts found that patients are entitled to a judicial hearing, and that the court determines competency and then makes a determination about treatment over objection based on a substituted judgment standard.

18. **A**

    Involuntary civil commitment is considered a significant deprivation of liberty in the United States. Persons involuntarily committed to a psychiatric hospital are unable to leave without medical approval, unable to choose their treating physician, and often unable to seek interhospital transfers. As a result of this significant deprivation of liberty, involuntarily committed patients are entitled to legal representation, either hired or court appointed, and a court hearing to determine the necessity of their involuntary commitment status.

19. **B**

    Although the patient's brother may be successful in having the feeding tube removed if he can present clear and convincing evidence of his brother's wish not to receive life-sustaining treatment (*Cruzan v. Director of Missouri Department of Mental Health*), family members cannot automatically make end-of-life decisions for incompetent relatives. It may be advisable to speak with multiple family members when, as a physician, you are considering a difficult clinical decision, but in this case, it is advisable to first consult the hospital risk management department to identify your legal and ethical responsibilities in the state in which you practice.

20. **D**

    The question of substituted judgement was considered in *Superintendent of Belchertown State School et al. v. Joseph Saikewicz*, Joseph Saikewicz had an extremely low IQ of 10 and had thus never been deemed legally competent. As a result of his incompetency, a guardian was put in charge of the decision to treat Saikewicz's leukemia with chemotherapy. Because Saikewicz was unable to comprehend the nature of the treatment and its many adverse side effects, the guardian recommended against administering chemotherapy. The small benefit of a limited extension of life was outweighed by the potential detriment of treatment. The case was heard by the Supreme Court of Massachusetts in order to establish a precedent on the question of substituted judgment (*Superintendent of Belchertown State School et al. v. Joseph Saikewicz*, Mass., 370 N.E.2d 417, 1977). The court agreed that extraordinary measures should not be used if the patient would not recover from the disease. The court also ruled that a person has a right to the preservation of his or her bodily integrity and can refuse medical invasion. The Supreme Court said that to presume that the incompetent person must always be subjected to what many rational and intelligent persons may decline is to downgrade the status of the incompetent person by placing a lesser value on his intrinsic human worth and vitality.

21. **B**

The U.S. Supreme Court case, *Baxstrom v. Herold*, held, in a unanimous decision, that equal protection "demands" that sentence-expiring convicts receive the same procedural safeguards that all others receive in the civil commitment process. The Court refused to specially classify mentally ill prisoners in order to avoid the standard procedural roadblocks to civil commitment. The case did not directly deal with board certification or any specific requirements of the certifying psychiatrists. The court made no finding of any prerequisite of community release since this would likely be too much of a public safety risk to be acceptable. Finally, the case did not address the burden of proof issue and it was not until 1979 that the Supreme Court established a burden of proof requirement for civil commitment in *Addington v. Texas*.

22. **B**

Youngberg v. Romeo was a U.S. Supreme Court case that addressed the due process rights of intellectually disabled, involuntarily committed individuals, including a right to freedom from restraint and to safety of confinement. There was disagreement at the circuit court level about what standard should be used in determining violations, since in some instances, restraints are necessary. The circuit court suggested "substantial necessity" and "compelling necessity"; however, the Supreme Court determined that it was "professional judgment."

SECTION III

Child and Adolescent Issues

CHAPTER 11

Child Abuse Reporting

SHAWN S. SIDHU AND ERAKA BATH

LANDEROS V. FLOOD, 551 P.2D 389 (1976)

Link to case: http://scholar.google.com/scholar_case?
case=3441539196251667835

Question: Can a physician who fails to diagnose battered child syndrome be found liable for subsequent injuries to the child?

Answer: Yes.

Gita Landeros, an 11-month-old baby, was taken by her mother to a local hospital for evaluation. A diagnostic workup by Dr. A. J. Flood revealed multiple bruises on baby Landeros's back and a leg fracture most commonly resulting from significant twisting force. She was treated and discharged back to the care of her mother. Shortly thereafter, baby Landeros presented again to another hospital where she was evaluated for multiple injuries, including an incompletely healed skull fracture and a left hand wound potentially severe enough to warrant amputation. She was diagnosed with battered child syndrome, and her mother and father were convicted of child abuse. The state-appointed guardian then filed a lawsuit against Dr. Flood for failure to identify physical injury secondary to maltreatment. The trial court dismissed the case, but on appeal, the Supreme Court of California ruled that the vast majority of physicians could have correctly diagnosed battered child syndrome and found in favor of baby Landeros. The court argued that the trial court erred in finding as a matter of law that Dr. Flood was not liable. A jury could reasonably have found that the

failure to diagnose the patient correctly and alert the proper authorities—
as mandated by California's reporting statute—ultimately resulted in harm
to the child.

PEOPLE V. STRITZINGER, 668 P.2D 738 (1983)

Link to case: http://scholar.google.com/scholar_case?
case=17744911620888675589

Question: Must a psychotherapist violate a patient's confidentiality if that
patient discloses evidence of child abuse that the therapist has already reported, based on the same information obtained from another source?

Answer: No.

Carl Stritzinger had been sexually abusing his daughter Sarah for 15 months
when Mrs. Stritzinger, his wife and Sarah's mother, learned of the molestation. Mrs. Stritzinger sought mental health services for both her husband
and her daughter with Dr. Walker, a psychologist. During the course of a
session, Sarah revealed that her father had sexually abused her. Pursuant
to mandated reporting statutes required by California law, Dr. Walker reported the incident to child protective services. After filing his report,
Dr. Walker was contacted by Deputy Buttell, in charge of investigating
these allegations. During their next scheduled session, Mr. Stritzinger
informed Dr. Walker of incriminating details regarding the allegations,
although no new information was revealed. Invoking psychotherapist–
patient privilege, Dr. Walker was hesitant to reveal content from his session and felt that he had already complied with his mandated reporting
duties by contacting child protective services. Deputy Buttell insisted that
Dr. Walker disclose content from the therapy session and referred to part
of the California Penal Code, claiming that it provided an exception to this
privilege based on the abuse-reporting requirements. Dr. Walker then gave
Deputy Buttell the information requested, and a transcript of that conversation was presented in Mr. Strizinger's criminal case, which ended with
his conviction. On appeal, the California Supreme Court found that the
trial court had erred in admitting evidence from Dr. Walker concerning the
substance of the consultation with Mr. Stritzinger. The court found that
because he had already reported the incident described by Sarah and did
not suspect any additional reportable activity, the obligation under the
child abuse reporting act was already met; and therefore, with reference
to the additional information, psychotherapist–patient privilege was still
in effect.

DESHANEY V. WINNEBAGO, 489 U.S. 189 (1989)

Link to case: http://scholar.google.com/scholar_case?
case=5543768239799414902

Question: Does a state have a constitutional obligation to protect a minor from violence perpetrated by a private citizen?

Answer: No.

Since the age of 1, Joshua DeShaney (a minor) was repeatedly abused and victimized by his father. These incidents resulted in several emergency room visits and investigations by social workers from the Department of Social Services (DSS) in Wisconsin. At each point in the investigation, the social workers did not feel that there was significant cause to remove Joshua from his father's home, so in lieu of placing Joshua in state custody, DSS made a voluntary agreement with the father that he would enroll Joshua in preschool and that he would enroll in parenting classes. The father failed to comply with these conditions, and in March 1984, Joshua's father beat him so badly that he was in a coma and suffered permanent and severe brain damage. Joshua and his mother filed suit in district court alleging that DSS had violated the Fourteenth Amendment by depriving Joshua of his liberty without due process by failing to remove Joshua from his father's custody. The district court granted summary judgment for DSS; the U.S. Court of Appeals also found in favor of DSS. The U.S. Supreme Court agreed that there is no violation of the U.S. Constitution when a governmental agency is aware that a child is being abused by a parent but fails to protect the child. The court found that the Due Process Clause refers to the state's responsibility against *state actions* and does not apply to the actions of *private* citizens, and that prior Court decisions found that the government had to protect life, liberty, and property only when the state had restricted an individual's liberty (e.g., civil commitment and criminal incarceration). The Court held that the Due Process Clause of the Fourteenth Amendment does not require a state to provide protection to the general public and that the state's due process duties are not so far-reaching as to impose duties to provide protection from violence by private actors.

CHAPTER 12

჻

Child Custody and
Parental Competencies

EILEEN P. RYAN

PAINTER V. BANNISTER, 140 N.W.2D 152 (1966)

Link to case: http://scholar.google.com/scholar_case?
case=15245255595862613942

Question: Is the standard for determining child custody based on the best
interests of the child?

Answer: Yes.

Harold Painter's wife died in a car accident when their son, Mark, was
5 years old. Mr. Painter requested that the maternal grandparents take
temporary custody of Mark. Mr. Painter then moved to California and
remarried. After 15 months, when he asked the grandparents to return
Mark, they refused. Although Mr. Painter was granted custody by the trial
court, the grandparents appealed to the Supreme Court of Iowa. The court
awarded custody to the grandparents, noting their "stable, dependable,
conventional, middle-class" environment as opposed to the father, who
they noted had a "bohemian" lifestyle, had held multiple jobs, and han-
dled money poorly. The court relied heavily on the testimony of a child psychologist who indicated that Mark's grandfather had replaced his father as
the primary "father figure" in Mark's life and also emphasized the importance of stability and continuity. The psychologist was concerned that the
bond between Mark and his father would not be strong enough to sustain
Mark through another wrenching loss and family transition. The court held

out the legal standard for determining custody as the best interests of the child, rather than the preference of the parent.

SANTOSKY V. KRAMER, 455 U.S. 745 (1982)

Link to case: http://caselaw.lp.findlaw.com/scripts/getcase.pl?navby=case& court=us&vol=455&page=745

Question: Is preponderance of the evidence the appropriate legal burden of proof for termination of parental rights?

Answer: No.

Two siblings, Tina and John Santosky, were temporarily removed from their biological parents for neglect. A third child was immediately removed at birth. The Department of Social Services (DSS) for Ulster County in New York moved for permanent termination of the parents' rights. The Santoskys had maintained contact with their children, but the family court determined that, even with public assistance, the Santoskys were unable to care for them. Permanent termination was ruled in the children's best interests at a disposition hearing by a preponderance of the evidence, New York's standard for the termination of parental rights in neglect cases. The Santoskys challenged the standard and Kramer, the commissioner of Ulster County DSS, claiming that the burden of proof for termination should be higher. The New York Supreme Court affirmed, but the New York Court of Appeals dismissed. The U.S. Supreme Court granted certiorari and found that the state's parens patriae interest in ensuring proper care for the child, and its interest in efficient administration of justice, need to be balanced against the "fundamental liberty" of the natural parents in maintaining their legal relationship to their child. Therefore, as with civil commitment (which also implicates liberty interests and mental health-related evidence), the near-equal allocation of risk between the parents and the state is unconstitutional. The Court ruled that the standard for terminating parental rights should be "clear and convincing evidence."

CHAPTER 13

Juvenile Rights

EILEEN P. RYAN AND ELIZABETH FORD

IN RE GAULT, 387 U.S. 1 (1967)

Link to case: http://caselaw.lp.findlaw.com/scripts/getcase.pl?navby=case&court=us&vol=387&page=1

Question: Are juvenile delinquents facing a loss of liberty entitled to similar procedural due process rights as adults charged with a crime?

Answer: Yes.

Gerald Gault was 15 years old when he and a friend were accused of making an obscene phone call to a neighbor, Mrs. Cook, allegedly commenting on her "bombers" and asking if her "cherries [were] ripe." Gerald was already on probation. He and his friend were picked up by the sheriff and brought to the Children's Detention Home in Gila County, Arizona. When Gerald's mother eventually learned of Gerald's arrest and went to the detention home, she learned that a hearing was scheduled for the next day in juvenile court. Notice about the hearing was not served on Gerald or his parents, no transcript of the hearing was made, no one was sworn in to testify, and Mrs. Cook, the complainant, was not present. At a second hearing, Mrs. Cook was again not present, despite Gerald's mother's request. A probation officer filed a report, which neither Gerald nor his parents saw, listing the charge as making lewd phone calls. Had Gerald been an adult, the maximum sentence he could have received was a $50 fine and 2 months in jail. The judge committed Gerald to a state training school until the age of 21.

Gerald's parents filed a petition for a writ of habeas corpus, which was dismissed by the Superior Court of Arizona and affirmed on appeal by the

Arizona Supreme Court. The U.S. Supreme Court heard the case and determined that although the juvenile justice had been historically based on trying to decriminalize juvenile delinquency, the potential loss of liberty associated with delinquency hearings demands procedural safeguards, similar to adults charged with a crime, under the Due Process Clause of the Fourteenth Amendment. Those safeguards include written notice, a right to counsel, and the right to confront witnesses.

GRAHAM V. FLORIDA, 560 U.S. 48 (2010)

Link to case: http://scholar.google.com/scholar_case?
case=6982366090819046045&hl=en

Question: Does the Eighth Amendment permit the sentencing of a juvenile offender to life without parole for committing a nonhomicide crime?

Answer: No.

Terrance Graham was placed on probation for a burglary and a robbery committed when he was 16 years old. Although Florida law allows discretion to prosecute 16- and 17-year-olds as adults for certain felonies, the judge in Mr. Graham's case withheld adjudication. Sometime later, now age 17, Mr. Graham was picked up for violating his probation by being involved in a robbery. Mr. Graham denied the robbery but admitted to fleeing from police officers after dropping his friend at the hospital following an alleged second robbery attempt. Under Florida law, the minimum sentence he could have received for the crimes was 5 years' imprisonment; the state recommended 30 years. A presentence report recommended 4 years. The trial court found Mr. Graham guilty of the earlier charges, noting Graham's "escalating pattern of criminal conduct," and sentenced him to the maximum sentence on each charge, amounting to life imprisonment without parole, since Florida had abolished its parole system. Mr. Graham filed a motion challenging his sentence under the Eighth Amendment; it was denied. Florida's First District Court of Appeal affirmed the sentence, and the Florida Supreme Court denied review. The U.S. Supreme Court heard the case and, based on the proportionality principle (whether the punishment is proportional to the offense), concluded that the Eighth Amendment prohibits sentences of life without parole for nonhomicide defendants younger than 18, and that states must provide such defendants with "some meaningful opportunity" for release.

MILLER V. ALABAMA, 567 U.S. 460 (2012)

Link to case: http://scholar.google.com/scholar_case?
case=6291421178853922648

Question: Does the Eighth Amendment permit mandatory sentencing of a
juvenile offender convicted of murder to life without parole?

Answer: No.

This U.S. Supreme Court decision represents the consolidation of two
cases, both involving 14-year-old defendants charged with murder. Evan
Miller, with a history of multiple placements in foster care as a result of
his mother's substance dependence and his stepfather's abuse, and with
a history of suicide attempts beginning at the age of 6 and prior juvenile
offenses, was involved in the murder of Cole Cannon following a drug deal
with Evan's mother. Kuntrell Jackson was involved in a robbery of a video
store that turned into a murder of the store clerk. Evan and Kuntrell were
charged and then convicted as adults, since both states (Alabama and
Arkansas, respectively) allowed prosecutorial discretion in moving the
cases to adult court. In both cases, existing state law required a minimum
sentence of life without parole for the crimes committed. Appeals courts
in both states affirmed the trial court findings and sentences. The U.S.
Supreme Court heard the cases and reversed the lower courts' findings,
using precedents in *Roper v. Simmons* and *Graham v. Florida*, among others,
as guidance. The Court found that the mandatory sentencing guidelines
for murder in Alabama and Arkansas, regardless of offender age, violated
the Eighth Amendment's ban on cruel and unusual punishment because
adolescents are, by their developmental immaturity, less culpable and
therefore less deserving of the most severe punishments. The Court did not
categorically ban imposition of such a sentence but required consideration
of the factors of youth in sentencing decisions.

CHAPTER 14

ᴄᐚᴐ

EAHCA (Education for All Handicapped Children Act); IDEA (Individuals with Disabilities Education Act)

SHAWN S. SIDHU

HENDRICK HUDSON BOARD OF EDUCATION V. ROWLEY, 458 U.S. 176 (1982)

Link to case: http://caselaw.lp.findlaw.com/scripts/getcase.pl?navby=case&court=us&vol=458&page=176

Question: Does the federal Education of the Handicapped Act (EAHCA) require schools to provide handicapped children "an opportunity to achieve full potential commensurate with the opportunity provided to other children?"

Answer: No.

Amy Rowley was a hearing-impaired student in New York who was otherwise bright and good at lip reading. Her parents, who were also both hearing impaired, met with the school a year prior to her starting kindergarten to discuss her education. In preparation, the school incorporated some technologies to help communicate with the family, and some staff members attended a course in sign language. Because Amy had some minimal residual hearing and was able to read lips well, she had success in kindergarten with the use of an FM transmitter. Prior to first grade, an Individualized Education Plan (IEP) meeting was held recommending placement in a mainstream classroom. The school also agreed to provide individual tutoring for 1 hour per day and speech therapy 3 hours a week. Amy's parents wanted her to also have a qualified sign language interpreter for all of her academic endeavors. The school, an independent examiner and the New York Commissioner of Education ultimately found this unnecessary because the student was doing well academically and functioning relatively independently. The EAHCA allows for judicial review and the parents brought suit in federal court. The district court and the U.S. Court of Appeals for the Second Circuit sided with Amy's parents; the case was appealed to the U.S. Supreme Court by the Hendrick Hudson Central School District. The Court ultimately reversed the judgment of the two lower courts, citing that the "free and appropriate public education" standard mandates that schools provide services that "permit the child to benefit from the instruction." The Court went on to write that the services provided by the school district "offered her [Amy] an educational opportunity substantially equal to that provided her non-handicapped classmates." While additional services may have allowed Amy to "maximally benefit" from her educational setting, she had achieved "adequate" academic success with the services already in place.

IRVING INDEPENDENT SCHOOL DISTRICT V. TATRO, 468 U.S. 883 (1984)

Link to case: http://caselaw.lp.findlaw.com/scripts/getcase.pl?navby=case&court=us&vol=468&page=883

Question: Is a child with spina bifida entitled to urinary catheterization during school hours under the Education of the Handicapped Act (EAHCA)?

Answer: Yes.

Amber Tatro was an 8-year-old student attending Irving Independent School District at the time of the case. She had spina bifida, which resulted in orthopedic pathology and speech abnormalities. The student was also unable to voluntarily empty her bladder completely at regular intervals due to a neurogenic bladder. Failure to empty her bladder would have resulted in damage to her kidneys, and therefore she required assistance emptying her bladder every 3 to 4 hours via clean intermittent catheterization (CIC). The catheterization procedure was a simple one that did not require medical training to complete, but rather could be completed by school nurses or any other trained adult. At Amber's IEP meeting, her parents requested that the school provide CIC services while Amber was at school; however, the school district refused on the grounds that CIC is a medical procedure and therefore should not be performed by school staff. Amber's parents brought the matter before the district court and state board of education. The district court ruled in favor of the school district, arguing that CIC is not a "related service" under the EAHCA because it was not directly related to education. The Court of Appeals for the Fifth Circuit reversed the ruling of the district court, stating that CIC was indeed a "related service," and further argued that not providing this service excluded Amber from access to basic educational services. The school district then brought the matter before the U.S. Supreme Court, which ruled in favor of Amber. The Court ruled that CIC is a "supportive service" without which Amber would not have been able to attend school, much less access special education. It ruled that CIC was not a "medical service," defined as "services provided by a licensed physician," because CIC can be performed by a school nurse or any other qualified adult who has received appropriate training.

CHAPTER 15

❀

Questions on Child and Adolescent Issues

QUESTIONS

1. The Education for All Handicapped Children Act (now known as the Individuals with Disabilities Education Act [IDEA]) was based on the expectation that all disabled children should have which of the following?
   A. Tuition waivers for more individualized private schools
   B. A free and appropriate public education
   C. Placement in a special education classroom
   D. Institutionalized education for the severely disabled
   E. Access to specialized nonpublic schools

2. The minimum standard of proof for the termination of parental rights is:
   A. Beyond a reasonable doubt
   B. Preponderance of the evidence
   C. Clear and convincing evidence
   D. More likely than not

3. In *Graham v. Florida*, the U.S. Supreme Court ruled that:
   A. The sentence of "life without parole" is prohibited for individuals who committed any offenses under the age of 18.
   B. The sentence of "life without parole" for individuals who commit nonhomicide crimes when under the age of 18 violates the Fourteenth Amendment's requirement for equal protection.

C. The sentence of "life without parole" for individuals who commit nonhomicide offenses when under the age of 18 violates the Eighth Amendment's prohibition on cruel and unusual punishment.

D. The sentence of "life without parole" for individuals who commit nonhomicide offenses when under the age of 18 violates both the Eighth and Fourteenth Amendments.

4. The importance of protecting psychotherapist–patient privilege is maintained by the following rationale:

A. The protection of privacy in a psychotherapist–patient relationship is thought to be important in establishing therapeutic alliance and to facilitate engagement in treatment.

B. Law enforcement needs supersede psychotherapist–patient privilege.

C. Mandated reporting of sexual abuse has a higher priority than reporting neglect.

D. Police can compel physicians and therapists to testify in cases of sexual abuse involving minors.

E. Psychotherapists must weigh maintaining patient privilege when public safety concerns exist around sexual abuse.

5. An 11-year-old student with chronic renal failure and end-stage kidney disease requires hemodialysis multiple times weekly. The patient's parents would like the child to have this service provided at school so as to minimally disrupt the educational process. Which of the following best describes the school's level of responsibility to perform the procedure based on the precedent set by *Irving Independent School District v. Tatro?*

A. Transport the student to and from the procedure.

B. Provide funding for the procedure.

C. The school has no responsibility for the procedure.

D. Send a private tutor with the student to the procedure.

E. Perform the procedure at the school.

6. The principle utilized in *Painter v. Bannister* for the determination of child custody was:

A. The tender years doctrine

B. The best interests of the child

C. Least detrimental alternative

D. Primary caregiver standard

7. Juvenile courts:
   A. Have been a fixture in the United States since colonial times
   B. Are a relatively recent invention, with the first juvenile court appearing in 1899 in Illinois
   C. Like criminal courts operate under the parens patriae principle
   D. Have always functioned similarly with respect to the roles and educations of attorneys and judges

8. The holdings of the U.S. Supreme Court in *Santosky v. Kramer* as they pertain to the termination of parental rights include:
   A. The primary interest of the state in parental termination hearings is the best interests of the child.
   B. While parents have an interest in preserving the family, the state has no such interest.
   C. There are shared interests in an accurate and just decision at fact-finding proceedings, and the near-equal allocation of risk between parents and the state is unconstitutional.
   D. The natural parents were not negligent, and the Santosky children should not have been removed.

9. When federal and state laws differ about a disabled student's entitlement to services, which of the following best summarizes the appropriate approach?
   A. It is permissible to follow the state law if it has fewer mandates than the federal law.
   B. Both laws must be put before a legal professional who is an expert in case law to establish the best next step.
   C. The parents can list their preference with regard to which law is followed based on the subsequent services to be provided.
   D. The state law applies when the state mandates services beyond federal requirements.
   E. The school district can choose the law that seems more applicable as long as it cites the reason for doing so.

10. Among the constitutional rights afforded juvenile defendants after *In re Gault* are:
    A. The right to an appeal
    B. The right to a jury trial
    C. The right to counsel
    D. The right to bail and a speedy trial

11. Implications of *Santosky v. Kramer* for children include:
    A. Child protective services will have a more difficult time investigating neglect and abuse allegations.
    B. Some children will not be removed from abusive or neglectful homes because it is more difficult to find clear and convincing evidence of abuse or neglect.
    C. More funding was made available for child protective service agencies around the country.
    D. Child protective services is able to remove children from abusive or neglectful homes more easily and efficiently than before.

12. Concepts underlying the philosophy of the juvenile court include:
    A. Closed proceedings and sealed records prevent discovery of procedural irregularities.
    B. The disposition should fit the offender rather than the offense in the interest of rehabilitation.
    C. Punishment as an extension of just desserts.
    D. Punishment is reserved for only the most severe and heinous of crimes, such as rape and murder.

13. A physician evaluates a child and is concerned about the potential for child abuse. The physician makes a report to child protective services, and the case is ultimately closed when no suspicious activity is found. The parents feel humiliated by the allegation and sue the physician for defamation and a violation of privacy. Which of the following most accurately represents the legal stance regarding this matter?
    A. Courts in most states tend to prioritize the rights of parents, and the physician is potentially liable.
    B. States vary greatly on this issue, and there is little national consensus on the matter.
    C. The outcomes of these cases are most dependent on the testimony of the child.
    D. Physicians who report in good faith are generally immune from liability for any damages.
    E. Parents are typically not allowed to bring suits against physicians for violations of privacy.

14. A clear and convincing standard for the termination of parental rights is justified because:
    A. Parental termination implicates a significant liberty interest, and parents who face removal of a child are often poor and uneducated and do not have the resources to oppose the state which may make it more likely with a preponderance of the evidence standard that errors will be made.

B. Parents have the right to reasonably discipline their children.

C. DSS does not give parents assistance in reestablishing a weakened parent–child bond.

D. A liberty issue is not at stake.

15. In *DeShaney v. Winnebago*, the main thrust of the ruling is based on the following principle:
    A. Due process protections are the foundation for mandated child abuse reporting statutes.
    B. The state has a duty to provide youth with adequate protection from all forms of abuse from parents.
    C. The state only has a duty to provide youth with protection from harm from state agents.
    D. The Due Process Clause protects citizens against state actions and those of private citizens.

16. In *Graham v. Florida*, the Supreme Court cited which of the following in support of its opinion?
    A. Juveniles are immature and have an underdeveloped sense of responsibility.
    B. Most jurisdictions that technically allow juveniles to receive a life sentence without parole only rarely impose such a sentence.
    C. Juveniles are more capable of change than adults.
    D. All of the above.

17. Which of the following is correct with respect to the Iowa Supreme Court's custody decision in *Painter v. Bannister*?
    A. Security and stability in the home are more important than intellectual stimulation in the development of a child.
    B. A parent's or caretaker's philosophy and way of life "within normal and proper limits" are irrelevant with respect to the determination of custody.
    C. The expert testimony of the child psychiatrist was afforded negligible weight.
    D. The child's relationship with his grandfather, which was stronger than that with his father, received little attention in the decision.

18. Which of the following is correct about sentencing guidelines for a 15-year-old convicted of capital murder in adult court?
    A. The fact finder is required to impose a minimum sentence of life without parole, although the death penalty can be considered.
    B. The fact finder is required to impose a minimum sentence of life without parole but cannot consider the death penalty.
    C. The fact finder cannot sentence the defendant to life without parole.

D. The fact finder must consider the impact of youth when imposing a sentence.

E. A 15-year-old cannot be tried in adult court.

19. Which of the following best justifies a breach in physician–patient confidentiality in cases of suspected child abuse?

A. Justice for the alleged perpetrator

B. The safety of the child at risk

C. Prevention of professional liability

D. The safety of the public at large

E. Physician acting as an agent of the state

ANSWERS

1. **B**

The EAHCA mandated that all handicapped children receive a "free appropriate public education." This term has continued to be applied in educational settings and, although vague, is the basis for many of today's educational standards. While some children spend time in special education classrooms and others go to specialized nonpublic schools, these accommodations do not apply to all disabled students and depend on individual and local district resources.

2. **C**

The minimum standard of proof for the termination of parental rights is clear and convincing evidence. In *Santosky v. Kramer*, the U.S. Supreme Court noted that parents faced with the irrevocable dissolution of their parental rights have a greater need for procedural protections than do parents resisting state involvement in ongoing family matters, such as temporarily removing children secondary to neglect.

3. **C**

In *Roper v. Simmons* (2005), the U.S. Supreme Court held that executing individuals under age 18 at the time of the offense was a violation of the Eighth Amendment's prohibition against cruel and unusual punishment. In *Graham v. Florida*, the majority opinion of the Court reaffirmed their reasoning, holding that juveniles were immature and therefore less culpable and less deserving of the most severe punishments. Neither case prohibited imposing the sentence of life without parole on individuals who commit murder before the age of 18.

4. **A**

   Law enforcement needs do not necessarily compel breeches in doctor–patient or psychotherapist–patient confidentiality. Regardless of the type, mandated reporters should report all child maltreatment to the appropriate authority if a reasonable suspicion exists. While a psychotherapist is indeed a mandated reporter of child abuse, the protection of privilege stems from the need to maintain treatment engagement and a therapeutic alliance, not public safety interests.

5. **C**

   Given that hemodialysis is a complicated medical procedure that employs the use of a dialysis machine and requires specialized training to administer, it would be considered a "medical service" rather than a "supportive service," and the school would not have any additional responsibility beyond common courtesy (observing the patient, alerting parents and authorities if the patient does not appear to be doing well, etc.). Funding should come from the patient's insurance or public aid. Of note, for nonmedical issues related to special education, the school may have to provide transportation services.

6. **B**

   In *Painter v. Bannister*, the Iowa Supreme Court concluded that remaining in the secure and stable custody of grandparents, rather than the unstable, but potentially more intellectually stimulating, custody of the father served the best interests of the child. Most jurisdictions determine custody on the basis of the best interests of the child standard, although considerable judicial discretion is allowed.

7. **B**

   The first juvenile court appeared in 1899 in Chicago, Illinois, and the concept grew in popularity. In juvenile court, the state as *parens patriae* would act as an advocate of youths, rather than as an adversary, and provide them with the help and treatment they required to overcome their youthful misdeeds. Due process was not considered to be necessary because the state was acting on behalf of the juvenile and therefore protection was unnecessary. Formal rules and procedures might hamper the court's mission and prescriptive "treatments." Prior to *Gault*, the key players in the juvenile court were social workers, mental health professionals, and probation officers. There was little law, and, therefore, little need for attorneys, and many of the judges were not legally trained. The most important question revolved around amenability to treatment.

8. **C**

Justice Blackmun in the majority opinion wrote that the Court expressed no opinion regarding the merits of the Santoskys' claims regarding their fitness for parenting the children who had been removed and noted that at "a hearing conducted under a constitutionally proper standard" (clear and convincing evidence, rather than preponderance of the evidence), "they may or may not prevail." The Court vacated the judgment of the New York Appellate Division and remanded the case for further proceedings. The "best interests of the child" standard was more clearly articulated in *Painter v. Bannister*.

9. **D**

With regard to the education of handicapped students, federal law sets a bare minimally acceptable standard. Many states may extend regulations beyond this bare minimum, but state law may not undercut the minimal standard set by the U.S. Congress or Supreme Court.

10. **C**

In re Gault's decision held that juveniles had the right to notice of charges, to counsel, to confrontation and cross-examination of witnesses, and to privilege against self-incrimination. Juveniles in juvenile court do not have the right to an appeal, a jury trial, a transcript of the proceedings, or the right to a speedy trial. Youths who are tried in adult court do have these rights.

11. **B**

Some child advocates have noted that by making termination of parental rights more difficult by raising the burden of proof, the Supreme Court decision in *Santosky v. Kramer* created a presumption against termination of parental rights, and that children have rights that do not necessary coincide with those of their parents or the state. The higher burden and proof may result in the already overstretched agencies charged with investigating abuse and neglect to have inadequate evidence to meet the increased burden; hence, more children will remain in neglectful homes.

12. **B**

Proceedings are closed and records sealed in juvenile court to avoid stigma and are in keeping with the benevolent nature of the court. Because the focus of the juvenile court is on rehabilitation and treatment rather than punishment, the disposition is tailored to the offender rather than the offense.

13. **D**

   While all of the answer choices in this question could technically be correct depending on the specific situation, the best answer is that doctors are generally protected when making decisions in the best interest of the child. Physicians may be held liable if the reporting is malicious, antagonistic, or otherwise unfounded. However, the law clearly favors reporting suspected abuse over withholding suspicions due to concerns about parental confidentiality. Potential penalties for not reporting suspected abuse are significantly greater than violations of confidentiality.

14. **A**

   In its decision, the U.S. Supreme Court noted that there was a liberty issue at stake in *Santosky v. Kramer*, and more substantial than the loss of money or property, where the standard of proof is preponderance of the evidence. The Court noted that the parents' interest in a termination proceeding is major (the loss of their children and family), and there is substantial risk of error involved if the standard used is preponderance of the evidence. Additionally, the government interest in favoring the preponderance of the evidence standard is slight. The Court's opinion also reflected the difficulty that poor, uneducated parents may have in mounting a defense against "[t]he State's ability to assemble its case" and referred to the state's "unusual ability to structure evidence," increasing the "risk of an erroneous fact finding," noting that DSS sought court orders denying the Santoskys visitation with their children, which if successful would have put them out of compliance with the Family Court Act's requirement for maintaining contact with their children.

15. **C**

   In *DeShaney v. Winnebago*, the court ruled that the Due Process Clause protects citizens against state action but *not* against the actions of private citizens. The state has a duty to provide youths with protection from harm from state agents only. State child abuse reporting requirements preempt physician–patient privilege. *Landeros v. Flood* relates to establishing battered child syndrome and is a foundational case in establishing mandated reporting of child abuse and neglect.

16. **D**

   In *Graham v. Florida* the Supreme Court utilized the same reasoning as in *Roper v. Simmons*. These include (1) juveniles' lack of maturity and underdeveloped sense of responsibility; (2) their increased susceptibility to negative influences and outside pressures, including peer pressure; and (3) their more malleable personalities, which are "not as well formed."

17. **A**

    While some of the biases revealed by the Iowa Supreme Court in *Painter v. Bannister* are often quoted, including his "artsy" father's "bohemian lifestyle," the court's opinion clearly indicates that the judges attempted to consider thoughtfully what was in the child's best interests and had an appreciation of the fact that the "divergent life patterns" of the father "seem[ed] to represent alternative normal adaptations." They attempted to contextualize the differences in life-style and the facts of the case as they applied to Mark Bannister. As is often the case in today's child custody disputes, the opinion of the expert witness in this case was given considerable weight. However, it is interesting to note that the trial court, which awarded custody to the father, dismissed the testimony of the expert, in part because it was "dismissive" of the role of the natural father. One of the factors given weight by the Supreme Court was that the psychologist opined that it was "very evident" that Mark considered his grandfather to be his father figure.

18. **D**

    According to *Miller v. Alabama*, trial courts must consider the contribution of youth (including developmental immaturity and diminished culpability) when sentencing juveniles who have been convicted of serious crimes (e.g., murder). Mandatory sentencing guidelines of life without parole for juveniles violate the Eighth Amendment, and therefore (A) and (B) are incorrect. However, there is still room for the fact finder to sentence a juvenile to life without parole if the factors of youth have been considered; (C) is therefore incorrect. Answer (E) is incorrect because adolescents in many jurisdictions can be tried in adult court for certain crimes.

19. **B**

    Answers B, C, and E may all be associated with a physician decision to breach confidentiality. For example, when quarantining an infectious patient, physicians are protecting the public at large and acting as an agent of the state. In these cases, the safety of individual patients may even take a back seat to that of the general public. However, in the case of child abuse, a breach of confidentiality is specifically intended to protect the child. Preventing liability should not in and of itself be the primary consideration, although appropriate clinical and legal decision-making mitigate potential liability.

SECTION IV

Tort Law

CHAPTER 16

༺

ADA and Disability Rights

HOWARD FORMAN, HEATHER ELLIS CUCOLO, AND MERRILL ROTTER

CARTER V. GENERAL MOTORS, 106 N.W. 2D 105 (1960)

Link to case: http://scholar.google.com/scholar_case?
case=1155130287709691700

Question: Are emotional disabilities compensable under workers' compensation even if they do not result from a direct physical injury or a single mentally disturbing event (e.g., seeing a coworker crushed to death)?

Answer: Yes.

James Carter was employed by General Motors (GM) and developed psychosis. Mr. Carter sought workers' compensation benefits. Medical testimony by Mr. Carter's treating psychiatrist stated that his psychosis resulted from emotional pressure encountered during the course of his daily work activities (assembly line work). The treating psychiatrist testified that, at some point, Mr. Carter's psychotic symptoms completely resolved, but that he could not return to the same type of employment because the pressures of the job might lead him to become psychotic again. The Michigan Workman's Compensation Appeals Board granted Mr. Carter benefits even though the psychosis resulted from "emotional pressures" rather than from a "single fortuitous event" such as a workplace accident. Also, the board granted benefits on an ongoing basis, having found that Mr. Carter could not return to work because of the risk of the return of psychotic symptoms. General Motors appealed the decision to the Michigan State Supreme Court. The court affirmed that although Mr. Carter became psychotic only while working at GM because of normal daily pressures combined with Mr. Carter's "predisposition to the development of a schizophrenic process," he was entitled to workers' compensation during the period of his psychosis. The Michigan State Supreme Court reversed the decision, holding that Mr. Carter was no longer entitled to benefits once his psychosis had resolved, because at that point he would return to being a person with the "predisposition" to develop psychosis.

CITY OF CLEBURNE, TEXAS V. CLEBURNE LIVING CENTER, 473 U.S. 432 (1985)

Link: https://caselaw.findlaw.com/us-supreme-court/473/432.html

Question: Does a regulation requiring a special permit for developmentally disabled adults violate the equal protection clause of the Fourteenth Amendment?

Answer: Yes.

In *City of Cleburne, Texas*, the city council of Cleburne denied a required and properly submitted special use permit to open a group home for 13 men and women with developmental disabilities. The proposed group home fell within the category of "[h]ospitals for the insane or feeble-minded, or alcoholic [*sic*] or drug addicts, or penal or correctional institutions" (at 436) and thus required the special use permit. The council's denial was premised on the assumption that neighboring property owners and elderly residents would be fearful of the developmentally disabled residents and that the intended group home occupants would be subjected to harassment by community members. Cleburne Living Center appealed the decision, alleging that the permit requirement violated the equal protection clause of the Fourteenth Amendment. The federal district court upheld the City of Cleburne's ordinance. Under the lowest level of scrutiny, the court found that the ordinance was rationally related to the city's interests. The Court of Appeals for the Fifth Circuit reversed the district court's finding and invalidated the ordinance because it did not further any important governmental interest. The City of Cleburne appealed to the U.S. Supreme Court. In a unanimous judgment, the Supreme Court held that the denial of the special use permit to Cleburne Living Centers, Inc. was premised on an irrational prejudice against the mentally retarded. The Court reasoned that "mere negative attitudes, or fear, unsubstantiated by factors which are properly cognizable in a zoning proceeding, are not permissible bases for treating a home for the mentally retarded differently from apartment houses, multiple dwellings, and the like." There being no rational basis for the special use permit, the requirement as applied to the proposed residence was invalidated as a violation of the equal protection clause of the Fourteenth Amendment. However, inasmuch as in this case the city failed to meet even the lowest standard for judicial review was clearly met, that is, rational basis, the Court declined to endorse a more exacting standard of judicial review, that is, strict scrutiny, which would have required demonstration of a compelling state interest to uphold legislation that differentiates one group of citizens from another, rather than merely a rational basis for the unequal treatment. The Fair Housing Amendments Act of 1988 (FHAA), barring discrimination in housing on the basis of disability and the Americans with Disability Act, passed in 1990, created the basis, under federal law, for higher levels of legal protection for individuals with developmental disabilities.

BRAGDON V. ABBOTT, 524 U.S. 624 (1998)

Link to case: http://scholar.google.com/scholar_case?
case=11295524924367699420

Question: Is HIV status a disability as defined by the American with Disabilities Act (ADA)?

Answer: Yes.

Sidney Abbott had asymptomatic HIV and went to her dentist to have a cavity filled. The dentist, Dr. Randon Bragdon, refused to perform the procedure unless it was done in a hospital, claiming that any other setting would pose a risk to him. Although Dr. Bragdon stated that he would not charge extra for his services, Ms. Abbott would have to pay any costs related to the use of the hospital's facility. The ADA defines a health care provider's office as a "place of public accommodation" covered by the act, but protections from the ADA may be set aside when the disabled individual "poses a direct threat to the health or safety of others." Ms. Abbott sued Dr. Bragdon on the ground that he violated the ADA because he discriminated against her on the basis of HIV, which she claimed met criteria as an ADA disability since it is a "physical impairment" that "substantially limits" a "major life activity" (i.e., her ability to reproduce and bear children). The district court and the U.S. Court of Appeals for the First Circuit both ruled in favor of Ms. Abbott, reasoning that (1) HIV infection (even when asymptomatic) is a disability, and (2) according to standards promulgated by the ADA, her HIV did not present any direct threat to Dr. Bragdon's health in his office. The U.S. Supreme Court agreed with the lower court decisions that

HIV is a disability, inasmuch as just having the infection impacted a major life activity (i.e., reproduction), but remanded the case to the appeals court for consideration of whether Dr. Bragdon had a reasonable claim that performing the procedure placed him at risk.

PENNSYLVANIA V. YESKEY, 524 U.S. 206 (1998)

Link to case: http://scholar.google.com/scholar_case?
case=3291537490094626018

Question: Does the ADA apply to people who are incarcerated in state prisons?

Answer: Yes.

Ronald Yeskey was sentenced to 18 to 36 months in Pennsylvania State Prison for drunken driving, escape, and resisting arrest. The sentencing court recommended that he be placed in Pennsylvania's motivational boot camp for first-time offenders. If Mr. Yeskey completed the boot camp successfully, he would only be incarcerated for a total of 6 months and then paroled. Mr. Yeskey was denied admission to the boot camp because he suffered from hypertension. He subsequently sued Pennsylvania's Department of Corrections, claiming it had violated the ADA by denying him the opportunity to participate in a program that could shorten his incarceration. The district court dismissed Yeskey's claim on the grounds that state prisons are not subject to the ADA. The U.S. Court of Appeals for the Third Circuit reversed this decision, and Pennsylvania appealed to the U.S. Supreme Court, arguing that the prison does not provide "benefits" as referenced by the ADA, and that the statute was intended to prevent the denial of disabled individuals from voluntary participation in services or programs. The U.S. Supreme Court affirmed the appellate decision and said that prisons do provide benefits, the statute did not presume voluntariness, and that despite the inherent loss of liberty, a prisoner could still voluntarily participate in programming. Therefore, Mr. Yeskey was indeed entitled to protection from discrimination despite being an inmate.

OLMSTEAD V. ZIMRING, 527 U.S. 581 (1999)

Link to case: http://caselaw.lp.findlaw.com/scripts/getcase.pl?navby=case&
court=us&vol=527&page=581#section1

Question: Does continued confinement of individuals with mental disabilities in hospitals beyond their clinical need for that level of care constitute discrimination under the ADA?

Answer: Yes.

Tommy Olmstead was the commissioner of the Georgia Department of Resources. Jonathan Zimring was a guardian ad litem for L.C., a mentally retarded woman with schizophrenia. L.C. was admitted to Georgia Regional Hospital for treatment of her psychiatric illness. After a period of inpatient treatment, it was determined by treating clinicians at the hospital that L.C. could safely be treated in a community-based program; however, she remained in the hospital pending placement in an appropriate outpatient program. She sued for relief pursuant to the ADA, arguing that her continued confinement was discriminatory in that she was precluded from access to the community equal to that of those without her disability. The U.S. Supreme Court agreed with Zimring that "unjustified segregation of persons with disabilities is a form of discrimination" and held that "states are required to place persons with mental disabilities in community settings when the State's treatment professionals have determined that community placement is appropriate . . . [and] is not opposed by the affected individual. However, the Court also added additional criteria, that is, that "the placement can be reasonably accommodated, taking into account the resources available to the State and the needs of others with mental disabilities." In appreciation of Georgia's concerns, the Court held that a state need not immediately transfer everyone to a community-based program but must have a mechanism by which people who are eligible to be transferred can be within a reasonable amount of time.

TOYOTA V. WILLIAMS, 534 U.S. 184 (2002)

Link to case: http://scholar.google.com/scholar_case?
case=3382304874478067867

Question: Does a disability that limits only specific work-related tasks qualify as a disability under the ADA?

Answer: No.

Ella Williams was a Toyota employee who suffered from carpal tunnel syndrome. Ms. Williams sued Toyota under the ADA, alleging that Toyota did not make "reasonable accommodations" for her disability. Toyota argued that carpal tunnel syndrome did not qualify as a disability because it did not substantially limit any of Ms. Williams's major life activities. The district court ruled in favor of Toyota, but the U.S. Court of Appeals for the Sixth Circuit reversed and ruled that Ms. Williams's inability to continue her work as a manual laborer represented an inability to perform a "major life activity." The U.S. Supreme Court reversed the appeals court decision, holding that the appellate court did not apply the proper standard for defining a disability because it failed to ask whether the condition prevented or restricted Ms. Williams from performing tasks that are of central importance to most people's daily lives. The Supreme Court held, "Merely having an impairment does not make one disabled for purposes of the ADA. Claimants also need to demonstrate that the impairment limits a major life activity." "Major life activities" refer to those activities that are central to daily life.

HARGRAVE V. VERMONT, 340 F.3D 27 (2003)

Link to case: http://scholar.google.com/scholar_case?case=6285186011968139170

Question: Does a validly executed durable power of attorney, which specifies preferred treatment alternatives, carry the same weight for individuals hospitalized for mental illnesses as for those without mental illness?

Answer: Yes.

Vermont law allowed individuals to execute a durable power of attorney (DPOA) for health care decisions in case they become incapacitated. Nancy Hargrave was civilly committed to Vermont State Hospital. She had previously executed a DPOA forbidding her agent from consenting to "any and all anti-psychotic, neuroleptic, psychotropic, or psychoactive medication." The hospital medicated Ms. Hargrave in a nonemergent situation. She sued, claiming that her DPOA was ignored because of her mental illness and that her mental illness rendered her disabled and thereby protected by the ADA. Vermont Act 114, which allowed the state to medicate a civilly committed individual even if the individual had a DPOA refusing treatment, had no corresponding mechanism for medication over objection for people who were only physically ill. The state argued that no corresponding mechanism was necessary, since mental illness in an involuntarily committed individual posed a "significant risk" and was not due protection by the ADA. The district court granted summary judgment in favor of Ms. Hargrave, stating that Vermont Act 114 singled out the mentally ill for discrimination and thus violated the ADA; the U.S. Court of Appeals for the Second Circuit upheld the holding.

U.S. V. GEORGIA, 546 U.S. 151 (2006)

Link to case: http://caselaw.lp.findlaw.com/scripts/getcase.pl?navby=case&
court=us&vol=546&page=151

Question: Can a disabled inmate in a state prison sue the state under Title
II of the ADA?

Answer: Yes.

Tony Goodman, a paraplegic inmate at Georgia State Prison in Reidsville,
sued the State of Georgia, claiming that he was being discriminated
against because of his disability in violation of the ADA. He alleged
that during his time in prison he was confined 23 hours a day in a cell
so narrow he could not turn his wheelchair around. He also alleged that
he was denied access to programming, medical services, and needed assistance with bathing and toileting. Georgia argued that it did not have
to accommodate Mr. Goodman because the ADA violated its state sovereignty under the Eleventh Amendment, which prohibits the federal
government from impinging on states' autonomy except as specifically
provided in the Constitution. The district court dismissed the case,
stating that "state sovereign immunity" barred Title II ADA claims. The
U.S. Court of Appeals for the Eleventh Circuit agreed about the ADA
claims but reversed the decision based on Eighth Amendment claims.
The U.S. Supreme Court then granted certiorari "to consider whether
Title II of the ADA validly abrogates state sovereign immunity" against
claims related to Fourteenth Amendment (equal protection) violations
and therefore allows a state prisoner to sue for money damages. The
Court concluded that in the ADA statute Congress had explicitly invoked
its "power to enforce, by appropriate legislation" the constitutional
guarantee of equal protection across states and that therefore the ADA
created a private cause of action against states for conduct that violates
the Fourteenth Amendment.

DISABILITY RIGHTS OF NEW JERSEY, INC. V. COMMISSIONER, NEW JERSEY DEPARTMENT OF HUMAN SERVICES, 796 F.3D 293 (2015)

Link to case: https://caselaw.findlaw.com/us-3rd-circuit/1709793.html

Question: Is New Jersey's nonjudicial process for forcible medication a violation of the ADA?

Answer: No.

Disability Rights New Jersey, Inc., an organization that advocated for the disabled, brought this action against the state and commissioner of the state Department of Human Services, in order to challenge the policy regulating the forcible medication of involuntarily committed persons in state psychiatric hospitals in nonemergency situations. The plaintiffs in *Disability Rights* were comprised of involuntary civilly committed patients and CEPP patients (Condition Extension Pending Placement, i.e., persons who no longer needed the hospital's services but were still confined awaiting appropriate alternative placement). The plaintiffs alleged that not having a judicial process as part of the hospital's forcible medication procedure was a violation of Title II of the Americans with Disabilities Act (ADA). According to hospital procedure, a decision to forcibly medicate someone was decided by a panel of hospital employees, some who were involved in the patient's treatment and others who were not. The court denied relief on the Title II argument, because the ADA does not guarantee that disabled people receive the same procedural treatment, when being cared for or treated in a hospital setting, as those who are not disabled. The Third Circuit did not consider whether the right to refuse medication could be considered a "service, program, or activity" protected by the ADA. As part of the same lawsuit, plaintiffs argued that the hospital procedure also violated the Due Process Clause of the Fourteenth Amendment. For this analysis, the Third Circuit differentiated between the involuntarily civilly committed and the CEPP patient, ruling that, due to the procedural nature of their confinement, CEPP patients are constitutionally entitled to a judicial process before being forcibly medicated, while the civilly committed patients are not.

SHEEHAN V. CITY OF SAN FRANCISCO, 135 S.CT. 1765 (2015)

Link: https://caselaw.findlaw.com/us-9th-circuit/1658065.html

Question 1: Did forced entry by police into the living quarters of a woman threatening violence and known to them to have a mental illness violate her Fourth Amendment right against unreasonable search and seizure?

Answer: No.

Question 2: Were the police required to find reasonable accommodations in assessing the need for forced entry by police into the living quarters of a person threatening violence and known to them to have a mental illness under the ADA?

Answer: Not answered.

Teresa Sheehan was a person with a mental illness who lived in a group home. During a periodic welfare check, police were called after a social worker became concerned that Sheehan was a danger to herself or others. Officers arrived to transport Sheehan to a 72-hour involuntary commitment hold and entered Sheehan's room without a warrant. Sheehan threatened the officers with a serrated bread knife and forced the officers to retreat outside of her residence. The responding officers called for backup, but instead of waiting, they decided to reenter Sheehan's room, the result of which led to Sheehan being pepper-sprayed and shot in her head, torso, arms, and pelvis.

Sheehan sued the officers and the city for violations of her Fourth Amendment right to be free from warrantless searches and seizures as well as violations of the Americans with Disabilities Act. The district court granted summary judgment in favor of the defendants, and Sheehan appealed. The U.S. Court of Appeals for the Ninth Circuit held that there were triable issues of material fact as to whether the officers failed to reasonably accommodate Sheehan's disability as required by the Americans with Disabilities Act.

The Court reiterated its long-held opinion that public officials are entitled to qualified immunity unless they have violated a clearly established constitutional or statutory right. In this case, the Fourth Amendment right against unreasonable searches and seizures was not violated by the officers' actions. Under Fourth Amendment precedent, law enforcement officers may enter a home or residence without a warrant in situations that constitute an emergency. In this case, the second entry still fell under the emergency exception because potential or imminent injury of the occupant continued to exist. Not only was the warrantless entry of the officers upheld, but the Court also found that the use of force employed by the officers was reasonable under the circumstances, despite the claim that multiple rounds were fired.

Because the attorney failed to address the Americans with Disabilities Act question at oral argument, the Court did not rule on the ADA issue in its opinion.

CHAPTER 17

✿

Civil Liability and Emotional Harm

AMAR MEHTA

DILLON V. LEGG, 441 P.2D 912 (1968)

Link to case: http://scholar.google.com/scholar_case?
case=1779068908894362158

Question: Does a person who suffers emotional injury but was not exposed
to actual physical injury have standing to sue for negligence?

Answer: Yes.

In 1964, Margery Dillon was crossing a street several yards behind two
of her daughters. David Legg was driving a car that struck and killed one
daughter. Ms. Dillon filed suit seeking compensation for her deceased
daughter, as well as damages for herself and her surviving daughter who
witnessed the accident.

Mr. Legg moved for a summary judgment on Ms. Dillon's claim of emotional suffering. Summary judgment was granted by the trial court with
reference Ms. Dillon's claim on the grounds that she was not in the "zone
of danger," or an area within which she was at risk of actual physical harm.
However, it was not granted with reference to the surviving daughter
who was closer to the accident and, therefore, in the "zone of danger." The
Supreme Court of California reversed the decision on appeal, describing
"the hopeless artificiality" of the rule by pointing out that "the area of
those exposed to *emotional* injury" is much broader, and "no distinction can
be drawn between physical and emotional injury." The court maintained a
standard of "reasonable foreseeability" and offered guidelines to take into
account factors such as whether a plaintiff was near the scene, whether his

or her shock was the result of directly observing the accident at the time, and whether he or she was closely related to the direct victim.

THING V. LA CHUSA, 771 P.2D 814 (1989)

Link to case: http://scholar.google.com/scholar_case?
case=4005949371237649225

Question: Is the "foreseeability" standard established by *Dillon v. Legg* too expansive?

Answer: Yes.

In 1980, James La Chusa was driving his car when he hit a boy named John Thing. John's sister quickly told their mother, Maria, who rushed over to the road and saw her injured son. Ms. Thing then sued Mr. La Chusa for emotional harm, alleging that his negligence caused the injury to John and was proximately responsible for her distress. Mr. La Chusa successfully requested a summary judgment from the trial court on the grounds that Ms. Thing had not witnessed the accident herself. The appellate court reversed that judgment, giving legal standing back to Ms. Thing. Finally, the Supreme Court of California ruled that the trial court had been correct, and that Ms. Thing could not establish such a claim. It laid out strict conditions necessary to recover for the negligent infliction of emotional distress, which had become too expansive and confusing since *Dillon v. Legg*. Instead of following a broad "foreseeability" standard, a plaintiff had to be closely related to the injury victim, had to be present for and aware of the "injury-producing event" at the time, and had to have suffered more emotional distress than a "disinterested witness."

CHAPTER 18

⌯⌯⌯

Clinical Practice Liability

BRYAN C. SHELBY, MERRILL ROTTER, AND
ELIZABETH FORD

ROY V. HARTOGS, 85 MISC. 2D 891 (1976)

Link to case: scholar.google.com/scholar_case?
case=17414302291314969766

Question: Does sexual intercourse between psychiatrist and patient constitute malpractice?

Answer: Yes.

From 1969 to 1970, Dr. Renatus Hartogs treated Julie Roy, during which
time he also engaged in sexual intercourse "as part of her prescribed
therapy." Shortly thereafter, Ms. Roy sued Dr. Hartogs, alleging that she
had been emotionally and mentally injured as a result of his improper
treatment. Dr. Hartogs lost at trial and was found liable for both compensatory and punitive damages. On appeal, the court noted that the general
right to sue for cases of seduction had been curtailed, but that this was a
malpractice case, in which the doctor had failed to treat his patient within
professionally acceptable standards. The court noted, however, that the
trial jury had gone too far in assuming that Dr. Hartogs had neither the
malicious intent nor level of recklessness necessary for punitive damages
and that given Ms. Roy's long-standing psychiatric condition prior to the
alleged malpractice, the award of $50,000 was excessive. The case was
remanded for a new trial limited to compensatory damages up to $25,000.

A concurring opinion cited Freud in noting that there is "common agreement of the harmful effects of sensual intimacies between patient and therapist."

AETNA V. MCCABE, 556 F. SUPP. 1342 (1983)

Link to case: http://scholar.google.com/scholar_case?case=14176085046214731005

Question: Is an insurance carrier responsible for covering alleged malpractice involving sexual relations between a physician and patient?

Answer: Yes.

Aetna, a malpractice insurance carrier, sought a declaration of noncoverage, arguing that the sexual relationship between Dr. Donald McCabe and Ms. Gale Greenberg (1) "did not arise out of professional services" and (2) constituted an "intentional tort" (as opposed to an accident); thus, punitive damages should not be paid by the insurer. Ms. Greenberg was in treatment with Dr. McCabe for asthma and anxiety. Dr. McCabe provided therapy and medication that was "either illicit or 'contraindicated.'" Their sexual relationship began after 6 months, and they eventually lived together. Dr. McCabe continued to prescribe medication throughout their relationship. At trial, there was testimony that Dr. McCabe's treatment and "mishandling" of the transference fell below professional standards. The jury found in favor of Aetna. On appeal, the court found that Aetna had represented Dr. McCabe throughout the trial and had not made the professional services argument, and so could not now argue that the sexual relationship was not covered by the policy. The court further noted that the policy did not explicitly exclude "intentional" behavior from coverage. Finally, the court found that Dr. McCabe should not be able to shield himself from the pain of punitive damages through insurance, and so those could not be covered by the policy.

MAZZA V. MEDICAL MUTUAL INSURANCE COMPANY OF NORTH CAROLINA, 319 S.E.2D 217 (1984)

Link to case: http://www.leagle.com/decision/1984536319SE2d217_1529

Question: Does public policy prohibit insurance coverage of punitive damages based on medical malpractice?

Answer: No.

Dr. Robert Huffaker was the treating psychiatrist of Jeffery Mazza, who alleged that Dr. Huffaker engaged in sexual intercourse with Mr. Mazza's estranged wife and abandoned him at a vulnerable time during treatment. Mr. Mazza sued Dr. Huffaker, claiming medical malpractice and other grounds for relief. Dr. Huffaker had an insurance policy in effect issued by Medical Mutual. At trial, Mr. Mazza was awarded $102,000 in compensatory and $500,000 in punitive damages, and the court further issued a declaratory judgment that, as written, the insurance contract obligated Medical Mutual to pay. On appeal, the North Carolina Supreme Court held that, while North Carolina law was silent on this question, other state courts had found that insurance contracts could be held to cover punitive damages. The court upheld Dr. Huffaker's acts as medical negligence and not as intentional acts. Furthermore, the court stated that punitive damages are available for acts that are not just intentional but also "wanton, reckless, malicious or oppressive." The terms of the Medical Mutual insurance contract were interpreted to be broad enough to cover the punitive damages based on Dr. Huffaker's medical negligence.

WICKLINE V. STATE, 192 CAL. APP. 3D 1630, 239 CAL RPTR 810 (2D DIST. 1986)

Link to case: http://scholar.google.com/scholar_case?
case=15274898154834148181

Question: Did California's third-party payer owe damages for harm caused by the application of a cost-containment program that affected a treating doctor's medical judgment?

Answer: No.

Lois Wickline was diagnosed with Leriche's syndrome, which could only be treated surgically. Mrs. Wickline's health insurance, Medi-Cal, authorized surgery and 10 days of hospitalization for her condition. She underwent several surgeries over those 10 days. Her treating physicians determined she needed 8 more days of hospitalization, but Medi-Cal's reviewers denied this request, and her treating doctors did not protest or appeal this decision. She was discharged but returned to the hospital with complications that resulted in the amputation of her right leg. Mrs. Wickline sued Med-Cal for damages. The jury found for Mrs. Wickline. On appeal, the California Court of Appeals held that Medi-Cal, as the third-party payer, was not liable because the treating physician went along with the shortened length of stay. Mrs. Wickline's doctors never protested or requested an administrative appeal of Medi-Cal's initial decision. Although the court did not decide in

Mrs. Wickline's favor in this case, it did note that third-party payers may be held liable in instances of design defects in the cost containment system or arbitrary decisions regarding care reimbursement.

WILSON V. BLUE CROSS OF SOUTHERN CALIFORNIA, 222 CAL. APP. 3D 660, 271 CAL RPTR 876 (2D DIST., 1990)

Link to case: http://scholar.google.com/scholar_case?case=16670556625035342312

Question: As a matter of law, are there triable issues of fact against an insurance company medical review if the attending physician did not make an appeal?

Answer: Yes.

Howard Wilson was admitted to a hospital for psychiatric treatment. His treating doctor believed he needed a 3- to 4-week inpatient admission. Ten days after admission, however, the patient's insurance company would not pay for any further inpatient care. Unable to self-pay, Mr. Wilson was discharged. Three weeks later he committed suicide. His estate brought suit against the defendant insurance company, Blue Cross and Blue Shield, and the utilization review company, Western Medical. The companies successfully filed for summary judgment citing *Wickline*, but Mr. Wilson's estate appealed. On appeal, the California Court of Appeals stated that *Wickline* was not applicable in this case because the discharge in *Wickline* met the standard of care as a matter of law, did not involve an insurance contract, and involved a cost-containment program established by state law. Furthermore, even though the treating physician did not appeal the insurance company review and ultimately made the decision to discharge the patient, as had been dispositive in *Wickline*, it was not considered critical in this case. *Wickline*'s language, according to the court, was characterized as dicta and not controlling. Mr. Wilson's estate was granted permission to continue the lawsuit at trial.

CHAPTER 19

Sexual Harassment

ANDREW P. LEVIN AND MERRILL ROTTER

MERITOR SAVINGS BANK V. VINSON, 477 U.S. 57 (1986)

Link to case: http://caselaw.lp.findlaw.com/scripts/getcase.pl?navby=case&
court=us&vol=477&page=57

Question: Does a finding of sexual harassment require that the employee be
subject to a quid pro quo linking the terms of employment to sexual favors?

Answer: No.

Over a 4-year period, Michelle Vinson worked her way up on merit from
teller to assistant branch manager at Meritor Bank under the supervision
of Sidney Taylor, one of the bank's vice presidents. After she was fired
due to excessive sick leave, she filed suit under Title VII, claiming that she
had been sexually harassed by Mr. Taylor (i.e., discriminated against on
the basis of her sex). She alleged that Mr. Taylor made sexual advances to
which she acquiesced for fear of losing her job and subjected her to de-
meaning fondling and comments in front of other employees. At trial the
district court found that Ms. Vinson had not been the victim of sexual
discrimination or sexual harassment because her relationship with Mr.
Taylor was a voluntary one having nothing to do with her advancement or
promotions. The U.S. Court of Appeals for the DC Circuit reversed, finding
that sexual harassment includes the creation of a hostile or offensive
work environment even when the terms and conditions of employment
are not contingent on sexual favors (i.e., quid pro quo harassment). The
U.S. Supreme Court upheld the court of appeals ruling, affirming the Equal
Employment Opportunity Commission's Guidance of 1980 that stated a

"hostile environment" violates Title VII. The Court also overruled the district court's finding that voluntariness negates a claim of harassment, instead defining the test as whether Mr. Taylor's advances were "unwelcome," while acknowledging that determining whether or not an advance is unwelcome "presents difficult problems of proof."

HARRIS V. FORKLIFT SYSTEMS, INC., 510 U.S. 17 (1993)

Link to case: http://scholar.google.com/scholar_case?
case=5109910086591041329

Question: For conduct to be actionable as "abusive work environment" harassment, must it seriously affect an employee's psychological well-being?

Answer: No.

Teresa Harris sued Forklift Systems, claiming that the conduct of the company's president, Charles Hardy, constituted "abusive work environment" harassment based on her gender in violation of Title VII of the Civil Rights Act of 1964. The magistrate found that Mr. Hardy made Ms. Harris the target of insults and sexual innuendoes in front of other employees. On several occasions Mr. Hardy asked Ms. Harris and other women to pick up objects he had thrown on the floor and get coins from his front pants pocket. Although the district court adopted the report of the magistrate and found that some of Mr. Hardy's conduct offended Ms. Harris and would be offensive to a reasonable woman, it ruled that it was not so severe as to affect her psychological well-being, nor did the court believe that Ms. Harris was subjectively so offended that she suffered injury. It thereby ruled that Ms. Harris had not been discriminated against under Title VII. After the U.S. Court of Appeals for the Sixth Circuit affirmed this ruling, the U.S. Supreme Court considered the case and reversed, stating succinctly, "Title VII comes into play before harassing conduct leads to a nervous breakdown." Further, "a discriminatorily abusive work environment, even one that does not seriously affect employees' psychological well-being, can and often will detract from the employee's job performance, discourage employees from remaining on the job, or keep them from advancing in their careers." The Court went on to reaffirm the *Meritor* standard that actionable conduct must create an "objectively hostile" work environment and must also be "subjectively" perceived by the victim as abusive.

ONCALE V. SUNDOWNER OFFSHORE SERVICES, INC.,
523 U.S. 75 (1998)

Link to case: http://scholar.google.com/scholar_case?
case=11566261664355830474

Question: Does abusive behavior between an employer and employee of the same sex qualify as discrimination under Title VII of the Civil Rights Act of 1964?

Answer: Yes.

Joseph Oncale worked in an eight-man crew on an oil rig in the Gulf of Mexico. On several occasions he was forcibly subjected to humiliating sex-related actions against him by some male coworkers in the presence of the rest of the crew and on one occasion was sexually assaulted by a male coworker who threatened him with rape. After complaints to supervisory personnel produced no remedial action, he quit, fearing he "would have been raped or forced to have sex." His discrimination suit in district court ended when the court granted summary judgment for the employer, finding that Title VII did not create a cause of action for harassment by same-sex coworkers, a ruling affirmed by the U.S. Court of Appeals for the Fifth Circuit. The U.S. Supreme Court reversed this decision, unanimously holding that workplace sexual harassment is actionable as sex discrimination under Title VII even if the harasser and the harassed are of the same sex. The Court relied on an earlier precedent in a case of racial discrimination that found that "because of the many facets of human motivation, it is unwise to presume as a matter of law that human beings of one definable group will not discriminate against other members of that group." The Court further held that the conduct "need not be motivated by sexual desire to support an inference of discrimination on the basis of sex." Instead, as already established in *Meritor* and *Harris*, the conduct must be so "objectively offensive" as to alter the "conditions" of the victim's employment.

CHAPTER 20

Questions on ADA and Disability Rights

QUESTIONS

1. According to *Olmstead v. Zimring*, every state-hospitalized patient is entitled to timely community care once stable. "Timely" was defined as:
   A. Within 1 year.
   B. The Court did not give guidance on the amount of time.
   C. At a reasonable pace.
   D. Within 10 years.
   E. All deliberate speed.

2. A physician working with any health care third-party payer should:
   A. Understand and be prepared to appeal benefit claim denials if it is determined such denial could harm the patient
   B. Understand that the physician may still be liable for adverse treatment decisions
   C. Understand that there is a continued duty to treat the patient despite adverse benefit determinations by a third-party payer
   D. All of the above

3. In the United States, a plaintiff can recover damages for the negligent infliction of emotional distress based on:
   A. The impact rule
   B. The zone of danger
   C. Reasonable foreseeability
   D. Standards that vary from state to state
   E. Direct observation

4. Which of the following is true about the role of sexual desire in cases of discrimination on the basis of sex?
   A. Sexual desire is a necessary element in determining the presence of discrimination.
   B. The victim's perception of the harasser's sexual desire is necessary.
   C. The conduct need not be motivated by sexual desire.
   D. Both the victim and the abuser must experience sexual desire.

5. A sexual relationship between a physician and a patient may be covered by malpractice insurance because:
   A. It is a side effect of psychotherapy.
   B. It is an occupational hazard for the psychotherapist.
   C. It is considered substandard clinical care.
   D. It is against the AMA ethical guidelines.
   E. It is against the APA ethical guidelines.

6. In *Hargrave v. Vermont*, Vermont Act 114, which allowed the state to override a durable power of attorney for a civilly committed individual, was found to violate Title II of the ADA because:
   A. The length of time that the individual had to be committed before the state could seek a court hearing for medication over objection was too short.
   B. Vermont Act 114 did not require a court order for medication over objection and thereby did not grant civilly committed individuals due process.
   C. There was no commensurate act allowing a person with physical illness to have his or her durable power of attorney overruled.
   D. Vermont Act 114 did not take into account emergency situations where medication over objection was needed to ensure the safety of people in the hospital.

7. How does an employee's response to sexual advances bear on a finding of sexual harassment?
   A. If she voluntarily participates, then she was not harassed.
   B. The response is not considered, only whether the advances were "unwelcome."
   C. An employee's repeated participation indicates it was acceptable.
   D. Acquiescence to sexual advances must be tied to an understanding that participation will result in advancement.
   E. All sexual contact between employees and supervisors qualifies as harassment.

8. The standards laid out regarding recovery for emotional harm in the case of *Thing v. La Chusa* (1989) state that the plaintiff must:
   A. Be a close relative, have witnessed the event, and have suffered emotional distress
   B. Have been in a position where he or she was at risk of harm, but not necessarily have suffered a physical impact
   C. Have been a direct victim rather than a bystander
   D. Have been partially responsible for the event himself or herself
   E. Have been a close relative of the defendant, mentally reconstructed the accident, and felt shock

9. "Reasonable foreseeability," as a policy regarding claims of negligent infliction of emotional damages, refers to:
   A. Whether the victim could have reasonably predicted the possibility of an accident, and therefore avoided it
   B. Whether a plaintiff could have reasonably seen a way to avoid the accident, and therefore shares liability due to contributory negligence
   C. Whether a defendant could have reasonably expected a negligent act to cause the resultant outcome, and therefore has a duty to the plaintiff
   D. Whether a judge could reasonably anticipate the outcome of a case, therefore resulting in a summary judgment
   E. Whether a lawyer could have reasonably calculated the amount of damages to be awarded, and therefore set his fee appropriately

10. According to *Mazza v. Medical Mutual Insurance Company of North Carolina*, punitive damages can be pursued from insurance companies for acts that are considered:
    A. Intentional
    B. Reckless
    C. Wanton
    D. Medical negligence
    E. All of the above

11. The Americans with Disabilities Act was signed into law in what year?
    A. 1934
    B. 1964
    C. 1990
    D. 2008

12. James Carter, an employee of General Motors, sought workers' compensation benefits because:
    A. His hand was crushed by the machinery he operated on the assembly line.
    B. He witnessed someone get crushed by a forklift and could no longer come to work without experiencing disturbing flashbacks.
    C. He had a psychotic illness, and the symptoms were unremitting, thus making it impossible for him to return to work.
    D. The work Mr. Carter was asked to perform caused him emotional stress that led to psychosis.

13. You are the defendant in a case regarding a tort claim for emotional harm as a result of your alleged negligence. If you lose, what penalties could you face?
    A. The death penalty
    B. Imprisonment
    C. Corporal punishment
    D. Monetary penalties
    E. There is no penalty for emotional harm.

14. A "hostile environment" violates Title VII of the Civil Rights Act of 1964 when it:
    A. Results in injury to the employee's physical health
    B. Results in injury to the employee's psychological health
    C. Alters the conditions of employment regardless of injury
    D. Enables the employer to exhibit frank hostility

15. Why did the U.S. Supreme Court overturn the appellate court decision which found in favor of Ms. Williams in her suit against Toyota?
    A. Wrist injuries are never serious enough to warrant protection under the ADA.
    B. The ADA does not protect against employment discrimination.
    C. Ms. Williams's impairment did not interfere with a "major life activity."
    D. Ms. Williams was found to be malingering.
    E. Ms. Williams had a factitious disorder.

16. An important factor in the *Wickline v. State* and *Wilson v. Blue Cross of Southern California* decisions was the physician's:
    A. Decision to appeal or not appeal a denied benefit claim
    B. Participation as an expert witness
    C. Credibility as a witness
    D. Membership on the applicable medical staff

17. *Dillon v. Legg* and *Thing v. La Chusa*, two cases involving requirements for seeking compensation regarding emotional harm, were decided for what jurisdiction?
    A. The State of New York
    B. The State of California
    C. Sacramento County
    D. The United States
    E. The United Nations

18. A defendant is responsible for negligently inflicting emotional harm only under certain circumstances. This is based on the concept of:
    A. Infinite liability
    B. Duty
    C. Malfeasance
    D. Tort
    E. Autonomy

19. Which of the following constitutes the test for an "objectively hostile" work environment?
    A. Descriptions available in peer-reviewed journals
    B. An expert's determination that the environment was hostile
    C. An environment that a "reasonable person" would find abusive or hostile
    D. The consensus of the workers in that environment

20. For an incident to be covered by malpractice insurance, it:
    A. Must be an accident
    B. Must be intentional
    C. May never be intentional
    D. Depends on the details of the policy

21. In *Roy v. Hartogs*, the plaintiff was able to recover for her emotional harm because:
    A. Her psychiatrist was a registered sex offender.
    B. The sexual contact was nonconsensual.
    C. The behavior at issue constituted improper treatment.
    D. She had not given informed consent.
    E. Seduction often leads to psychological harm.

22. In the *Disability Rights New Jersey, Inc.* case, CEPP patients are persons who:
    A. Are not covered under Title II of the ADA
    B. No longer need the hospital's services but are still confined awaiting appropriate alternative placement

   C. Have the right to refuse medication because that right is considered a "service, program, or activity" protected by the ADA

   D. Are a protected class under the ADA

23. In *Sheehan v. City of San Francisco* the Court declined to answer whether police were required to find reasonable accommodations during a forced entry into the living quarters of a person threatening violence and known to have a mental illness under the ADA. With consideration of the other ADA cases in the chapter, which of the below accommodations do you think that law enforcement does not need to provide?

   A. An accommodation when interrogating witnesses

   B. An accommodation when providing emergency medical services

   C. An accommodation when receiving citizen complaints

   D. An accommodation when enforcing a criminal law relating to an individual's current use or possession of illegal drugs

ANSWERS

1. **C**

   To satisfy the court ruling, the State of Georgia would have to maintain a list of people to be transferred that moved at a "reasonable pace." The rate "all deliberate speed" comes from the landmark *Brown v. Board of Education* decision concerning school desegregation.

2. **D**

   A physician should be prepared to appeal adverse benefit determinations of a patient's insurance or utilization reviewer if the physician believes that continued care is medically necessary. A physician still may be liable for failure to pursue an appeal. A physician generally has a duty to continue to treat a patient until the patient is stable and can be safely referred, even if continued benefits are denied.

3. **D**

   In the United States, each state has different criteria regarding a plaintiff's standing to sue for the negligent infliction of emotional distress. Some outdated standards include the impact rule (physical contact was required) and the zone of danger (an area in which a person was at risk of physical harm). A standard overturned in California but still used in some other jurisdictions is foreseeability (whether a defendant could have reasonably expected his actions to have had the resulting consequences). In *Thing v. La Chusa*, California adopted a set of standards that include whether the plaintiff is a close relative of the victim, directly observed the accident, and suffered emotional distress as a result.

4. **C**

   In *Oncale v. Sundowner Offshore Services*, the U.S. Supreme Court observed that although sexual harassment cases typically involve implicit or explicit proposals of sexual activity, the conduct "need not be motivated by sexual desire to support an inference of discrimination on the basis of sex." A trier of fact may, for instance, find discrimination when the harasser is motivated by general hostility toward the victim on the basis of her gender, even if the harasser and the victim are the same gender.

5. **C**

   Challenging emotional states and potential boundary violations are well-known risks of intensive psychotherapy for both therapists and patients. The AMA guidelines prohibit sexual relationships with active patients. The APA guidelines prohibit sexual relationships with both active and former patients. However, malpractice is not bound by any of these clinical or ethical standards. Malpractice ultimately is based on whether the clinical treatment fell below the accepted standard of care in the community.

6. **C**

   The central principle of the ruling in *Hargrave v. Vermont* is that Act 114 allowed for the overruling of the durable power of attorney for a mentally ill civilly committed individual but did not do so for a person with only physical illness. The length of time to seek a court order was 45 days, but this was not an issue in the court's decision (A). Act 114 did require a court order for medication over objection (B). The state hospital had the right to medicate over objection in emergency situations and therefore had nothing to do with Act 114 (D).

7. **B**

   In *Meritor Savings Bank v. Vinson*, the plaintiff participated in sexual activity with her supervisor multiple times over the course of 4 years. Although she stated that she did this out of fear of losing her job, the district court characterized her participation as "voluntary" because she did not resist and based the rejection of her claim in part on her willing participation. The U.S. Supreme Court ruled that voluntariness was not the central issue, instead defining the test as whether the advances were "unwelcome." Under this definition, not all sexual activity between an employee and a coworker or supervisor would qualify as harassment.

8. **A**

In *Thing v. La Chusa*, the Supreme Court of California further defined the conditions that had been suggested in *Dillon v. Legg*. The court required that to have standing to seek damages for emotional harm, a plaintiff must be a close relative of the victim, have witnessed the event, and have suffered emotional distress. *Dillon v. Legg* had overturned *Amaya v. Home Ice, Fuel & Supply Co.* (1963), which stated that a plaintiff had to have been in a position where he or she was at actual risk of harm (the "zone of danger"). Option (E) is a combination of nonsensical propositions (that the plaintiff had been a close relative of the defendant).

9. **C**

In the case of *Dillon v. Legg*, reasonable foreseeability refers to whether or not a defendant could have reasonably expected a negligent act to cause the resultant outcome. If so, then the negligent actor had a duty to the plaintiff. A victim's ability to avoid an accident does not obviate the duty of others to avoid acting in a negligent manner. *Dillon* states that if the defendant is found not to be primarily liable due to the contributory negligence of the plaintiff, then that plaintiff cannot recover for emotional trauma; however, that is not what is meant by reasonable foreseeability. The ability of a judge to anticipate the outcome of a case does not in itself allow him or her to make a summary judgment, and, in any case, it has nothing to do with the term in question. Lawyer's fees also bear no relation to the term.

10. **E**

In this case, the court was concerned with the issue of whether it was against public policy for an insurer to pay punitive damages for medical negligence of a physician under an insurance policy. The holding in the case illustrated that a policy may be construed to require the payment of punitive damages, and punitive damages may include not only intentional acts but also acts that are considered reckless or wanton. *Mazza v. Medical Mutual Insurance Company of North Carolina* makes clear that it is not, as a matter of law, against public policy for insurance contracts to cover these damages.

11. **C**

In 1934, the Communications Act was passed and called for affordable communications technology to be made available to all people in the United States. Title IV of the ADA required that telecommunications options be made available for the disabled. The Civil Rights Act of 1964 made discrimination based on race, religion, gender, and national origin illegal. In 2008, President George W. Bush passed the ADA

Amendments Act into law, further extending some of the protections of the original act, which was signed into law by President George H. W. Bush in 1990.

12. **D**

Someone does not need to suffer a physical injury on the job to receive workers' compensation (A). It does not need to be a single horrific event that causes the mental illness for someone to be able to receive workers' compensation but can actually just be mental illness due to the daily routine demands of the job, as was the case with Mr. Carter (B). Mr. Carter's psychosis actually went into full remission (C). The Michigan State Supreme Court ruled that Mr. Carter was not entitled to workers' compensation during periods of remission because at that point he was only predisposed to something that would interfere with his ability to work.

13. **D**

A tort claim is, by definition, governed by civil law. Capital punishment and imprisonment are possible penalties only under criminal law; corporal punishment, or the deliberate infliction of pain as a form of discipline, occurs mostly in the legal context of child abuse. Civil cases can result in fines or financial compensation and may also result in actions by organizations other than the court (such as official censures or the revocation of privileges). If emotional harm is proved, penalties are certainly possible.

14. **C**

In both *Meritor Savings Bank v. Vinson* and *Harris v. Forklift Systems, Inc.*, the U.S. Supreme Court stated that a "hostile environment" exists when discrimination is "sufficiently severe and pervasive" so as to alter the conditions of employment. In many instances, plaintiffs claim that the hostile environment resulted in injury to their physical or psychological health, and experts are asked to opine regarding the extent of those damages. But the Supreme Court ruled in *Harris* that "Title VII comes into play before harassing conduct leads to a nervous breakdown." In other words, the existence of a hostile environment alone is sufficient to qualify as discrimination regardless of whether the plaintiff experienced additional injury to physical or psychological well-being.

15. **C**

Despite having carpal tunnel syndrome, Ms. Williams retained the ability to perform most activities of daily living. It appeared as though her only limitation was being able to continue working as a manual laborer. There is no class of injury or illness that is not open to ADA protection; it depends on the effects of the condition (A). Title I of the ADA specifically prohibits discrimination in employment on the basis of disability (B). There is nothing to suggest Ms. Williams was malingering or that her carpal tunnel syndrome was factitious (D, E).

16. **A**

The *Wickline* and *Wilson* decisions involved fact patterns where the physician did not appeal an insurance adverse benefit determination. This fact was more dispositive for the underlying issue in the *Wickline* case than in the *Wilson* case, but both cases illustrate the role of the physician's final decision. The court held in *Wilson* that the physician's failure to place an appeal did not relieve the third-party reviewer of the potential for liability.

17. **B**

Though the legal reasoning described in the opinions has served as the basis for many other state policies, the landmark cases regarding negligent infliction of emotional damages were decided by the Supreme Court of California and therefore apply only to the State of California. *Dillon v. Legg* initially started in the county of Sacramento, but the legal precedent was set for the entire state. New York has a separate legal system, though it has been informed by the debate surrounding the decisions of other states. The U.S. Supreme Court has not set a policy for the entire country to follow, and the United Nations is an international organization consisting of nearly 200 countries.

18. **B**

Duty is a concept referring to a legal obligation and only exists between two parties under specifically defined circumstances. Infinite liability (the potential for anyone to sue for damages stemming from any particular negligent act) is a problem that the courts attempt to avoid by placing restrictions on who has legal standing to bring a lawsuit. Malfeasance is an intentional wrongful act, often in an official context. Tort also means an injury or wrongful act, but it may be intentional or accidental. Autonomy is an unrelated concept regarding the ability of rational people to make informed decisions for themselves.

19. **C**

In determining whether a work environment is "objectively hostile," the fact finder must consider how a "reasonable person" would react under similar circumstances. In *Harris v. Forklift Systems, Inc.*, the U.S. Supreme Court cited several elements that might be used to define such an environment, including discriminatory intimidation, ridicule, and insult, as well as the environment's impact on an employee's performance, desire to advance, and motivation to stay on the job. Despite these signposts, the determination rests on the "reasonable person." Attorneys for both plaintiffs and defendants often attempt to introduce expert testimony to define this standard, but courts are likely to limit the role an expert can play in defining the reactions of a "reasonable person," leaving this up to the jury.

20. **D**

Cases of negligence are ones in which the harm caused was not intended. However, that is different from whether or not the action itself was intentional as opposed to an accident. In *Aetna v. McCabe*, the court noted that, in general, behavior can be considered malpractice whether it was accidental or intentional, but in this case the critical fact was that Dr. McCabe's policy did not specifically exclude intentional actions from coverage.

21. **C**

This case was treated as a pure malpractice case in which the sexual contact between psychiatrist and patient was deemed improper and below accepted professional standards. Dr. Hartogs was not a sexual offender, and there was no allegation that the patient had been coerced or uninformed. The court noted that the right to recover a sum of money for seduction as a general matter had been abolished, but that this case was one of malpractice, not seduction per se.

22. **B**

CEPP stands for Condition Extension Pending Placement, that is, persons who no longer meet the criteria for involuntary civil commitment but are still confined because the appropriate alternative placement has not been located and approved by the court.

23. **D**

Title II of the ADA prohibits discrimination against people with disabilities in state and local governments services, programs, and employment. Law enforcement agencies are covered because they are programs of state or local governments, regardless of whether they receive federal grants or other federal funds. The ADA affects virtually everything that officers and deputies do, including receiving citizen complaints; interrogating witnesses; arresting, booking, and holding suspects; operating telephone (911) emergency centers; providing emergency medical services; enforcing laws; and other duties. Answer "D" is correct because nothing in the ADA prevents officers and deputies from enforcing criminal laws relating to an individual's current use or possession of illegal drugs.

SECTION V

Criminal Law and Incarceration

CHAPTER 21

Criminal Procedure

MICHAEL GREENSPAN, AMAR MEHTA, MERRILL ROTTER, AND JEREMY COLLEY

ROBINSON V. CALIFORNIA, 370 U.S. 660 (1962)

Link to case: http://caselaw.lp.findlaw.com/scripts/getcase.pl?navby=case&court=us&vol=370&page=660

Question: Is a California statute making the status of drug addiction a crime unconstitutional?

Answer: Yes.

A California statute in 1962 made it a misdemeanor crime to "be addicted to the use of narcotics," further defined at trial as "a status or condition and not an act." Police officers in Los Angeles stopped Lawrence Robinson and observed track marks on his arms that they believed to be from intravenous drug abuse (Mr. Robinson claimed they were the result of an allergic condition). He was not intoxicated or withdrawing at the time and was not acting in a disruptive or antisocial manner. He was found guilty, and the verdict was affirmed on appeal. The case was then appealed to the U.S. Supreme Court for inflicting a "cruel and unusual punishment" in violation of the Eighth Amendment as applicable to the states through the Fourteenth Amendment. The Court agreed that the Eighth Amendment was applicable to the states, and it reviewed prior rulings supporting that "evolving standards of decency" should govern the definition of what would constitute "cruel and unusual punishment." The Court applied a proportionality analysis, finding that a brief imprisonment in itself was neither cruel nor unusual, but "even one day in prison would be a cruel and unusual punishment for the 'crime' of having a common cold." It was also noted that addiction could even occur "innocently or involuntarily," such as by exposure in utero or starting with a legitimate prescription. The statute was found unconstitutional, and the decision was reversed.

MIRANDA V. ARIZONA, 384 U.S. 436 (1966)

Link to case: http://caselaw.lp.findlaw.com/scripts/getcase.pl?navby=case& court=us&vol=384&page=436

Question: Are police required to inform a suspect of his or her rights to re-main silent and to have an attorney present?

Answer: Yes.

In 1963, Ernesto Miranda was arrested for kidnapping and rape. At trial, his attorney objected to the admission of his confession, contending that it was not voluntary. The objection was overruled, and Mr. Miranda was convicted. Upon arrest, Mr. Miranda had signed a confession that included a statement as to its voluntariness and with "full knowledge of my legal rights." However, he had not been explicitly advised by the police of his right to counsel or his right to remain silent. The Arizona Supreme Court upheld the conviction, and Mr. Miranda appealed to the U.S. Supreme Court, asserting that his Fifth and Sixth Amendment rights had been violated. The Court ruled that due to the inherently coercive nature of cus-todial interrogation, a suspect must be "clearly informed" of his rights and must explicitly waive them.

POWELL V. TEXAS, 392 U.S. 514 (1968)

Link to case: http://caselaw.lp.findlaw.com/scripts/getcase.pl?navby=case& court=us&vol=392&page=514

Question: Can public intoxication be treated as a crime if it is a result of alcoholism?

Answer: Yes.

A Texas statute in 1968 made it a crime, punishable by a fine, to "be found in a state of intoxication in a public place." Leroy Powell was arrested and found guilty of public intoxication in Austin and appealed to a county court. He argued that chronic alcoholism was a disease, and to punish someone criminally for suffering from a disease would be "cruel and unusual punishment" in violation of the Eighth Amendment, as applicable to the states through the Fourteenth Amendment (as decided in *Robinson v. California*). A new trial was held, and Mr. Powell was again found guilty. When he appealed to the U.S. Supreme Court, the resulting opinion included a review of the "disease" concept of alcoholism, as well as the "substantial disagreement within the medical profession" regarding its definitions and limitations. Medical testimony noted that "these individuals have a compulsion . . . while not completely overpowering, [it is] an exceedingly strong influence," and the Court decided that there was not enough clarity to remove responsibility. The guilty verdict was upheld on the grounds that Mr. Powell was not convicted for the status of being an alcoholic but rather for the act of being intoxicated in public at a specific time.

NORTH CAROLINA V. ALFORD, 400 U.S. 25 (1970)

Link to case: http://scholar.google.com/scholar_case?case=14055791673999770436

Question: Can a defendant plead guilty even though he maintains his innocence?

Answer: Yes.

In 1963, Henry Alford was indicted for first-degree murder, a charge carrying a potential death penalty in North Carolina. Faced with strong evidence of guilt, along with state procedure that allowed for a mitigation of punishment to life imprisonment with a guilty plea (as opposed to a jury conviction), Mr. Alford entered a guilty plea. On the stand, Mr. Alford stated that he was entering his plea only to avoid the death penalty, saying, "I'm not guilty, but I plead guilty." Following his plea, while incarcerated, Mr. Alford sought postconviction relief (first at the state level and later in the federal court of appeals) and failed in several jurisdictions, wherein his plea was felt to be a "voluntary and intelligent choice." In 1967, the Fourth Circuit Court of Appeals reversed the guilty plea, finding it to be involuntary because its principal motivation was fear of the death penalty. In a 6–3 holding, the U.S. Supreme Court reversed this decision. Despite Mr. Alford's claim of innocence, the Court felt that (1) the strong evidence supporting his guilt and (2) his representation by competent counsel resulted in a valid guilty plea. The fear of the death penalty, in and of itself, is not adequately coercive to invalidate a guilty plea within the meaning of the Fifth Amendment.

COLORADO V. CONNELLY, 479 U.S. 157 (1986)

Link to case: http://scholar.google.com/scholar_case?
case=13661442250005953902

Question: Is coercive police activity required for a finding of lack of voluntariness of a confession?

Answer: Yes.

On August 18, 1983, Francis Connelly approached a police officer in Denver, Colorado, and stated that he had committed a murder and wanted to confess. The police officer provided a *Miranda* warning and later stated that he did not believe Mr. Connelly to be clearly under the influence of substances or mentally ill at the time of the confession. The next morning, however, when questioned by the public defender, Mr. Connelly appeared confused and stated that he had confessed as a result of auditory hallucinations. Following restoration for lack of competence to stand trial, the Colorado trial court suppressed the confession, finding that it was not the product of a defendant's "rational intellect and free will" (citing *Townsend v. Sain* [1963], an earlier U.S. Supreme Court decision). The Colorado Supreme Court affirmed this on initial appeal. In a 7–2 holding, the U.S. Supreme Court reversed the decision, holding that coercive police activity is *required* to allow the suppression of a confession based on violation of the Due Process Clause of the Fourteenth Amendment. The Court allowed that mental illness is relevant to a defendant's susceptibility to state coercion, but that such illness alone and its effect on "voluntariness" do not constitute a due process violation.

COMMONWEALTH OF MASSACHUSETTS V. ELDRED, 480 MASS. 90 (2018)

Link to case: https://law.justia.com/cases/massachusetts/supreme-court/
2018/sjc-12279.html

Question: May a judge require that a person remain drug-free as a condition of probation, if she suffers from an addiction?

Answer: Yes.

In the summer of 2016, Julie Elred, an opioid addict, plead guilty to stealing $250 worth of jewelry, which she sold to buy drugs. The trial judged imposed a 1-year probation, the conditions of which were that she attend substance abuse treatment, submit to random urine drug screens, and remain drug-free. In September, Ms. Eldred tested positive for fentanyl. Her probation officer attempted to secure admission for Ms. Eldred to an inpatient drug rehabilitation facility but was not able to do so immediately. Ms. Eldred was held in jail for 10 days to await a full hearing regarding whether or not she violated her probation, and as a result of that hearing, was transferred to the rehabilitation facility by the order of the judge.

Ms. Eldred appealed her violation, claiming that her addiction rendered her incapable of remaining drug-free. The Massachusetts Supreme Court granted certiorari.

The Court ruled that an addict's conditions of parole can include abstinence, relying heavily on the argument that judges, in the context of probation, have considerable flexibility in establishing its terms, tailored to the individual, so long as "the conditions are reasonably related to the goals of sentencing and probation." Moreover, the Court clarified that punishment imposed for a violation of the terms of probation are not for the violation itself, per se, but for the offense for which probation was granted—in other words, in this case, the act to be punished was stealing, not drug use.

To this end, the Court side-stepped the issue of whether or not violating a probationer for failure to abstain constituted cruel and unusual punishment, in the spirit of *Robinson v. California*, which recognized that "addiction is a status that cannot be criminalized." In addition, in this case, Eldred had clearly used drugs and had not solely met diagnostic criteria for an addiction. The Court was careful to say that "the appellate record before the court is inadequate to determine whether SUD (substance use disorder) affects the brain in such a way that certain individuals cannot control their drug use."

CHAPTER 22

Criminal Competencies

MATTHEW W. GROVER, HEATHER ELLIS CUCOLO,
AND MERRILL ROTTER

DUSKY V. U.S. 362 U.S. 402 (1960)

Link to case: http://scholar.google.com/scholar_case?
case=2877494138671044176

Question: Is basic knowledge about one's charges enough to be competent
to stand trial?

Answer: No.

Milton Dusky was a 33-year-old man diagnosed with schizophrenia when
he was charged—along with two juvenile codefendants—of abducting and
raping a teenage girl. His attorney raised the issue of his competence to
stand trial, and Mr. Dusky was hospitalized for 4 months at a federal hospital for examination. The competency report noted that he was not able to
understand the legal proceedings against him, nor could he assist counsel.
One expert testified that he had difficulty with reality testing and was suspicious. The trial judge in the U.S. District Court in Missouri found him
competent to stand trial, noting that he was oriented to time and place, had
some recollection of events, and appeared to be able to assist counsel. Mr.
Dusky was convicted and sentenced to 45 years. The U.S. Court of Appeals,
Eighth Circuit, affirmed his conviction. The U.S. Supreme Court reversed
and held that the record did not sufficiently support the finding of competency to stand trial. While Mr. Dusky understood the basic elements of the
court proceedings and the charges, he was unable to assist counsel due to
his psychosis. The court held that the test of a defendant's competency to

stand trial is "whether he has sufficient present ability to consult with his lawyer with a reasonable degree of rational understanding—and whether he has a rational as well as factual understanding of the proceedings against him."

WILSON V. U.S. 391 F.2D 460 (1968)

Link to case: http://openjurist.org/391/f2d/460/wilson-v-united-states

Question: Must permanent retrograde amnesia render a defendant incompetent to stand trial?

Answer: No.

On October 2, 1964, Robert Wilson and his partner carjacked a man at gunpoint and robbed a pharmacy. As a result of the ensuing high-speed chase with a police cruiser, the defendants crashed the car into a tree. The partner died, but Mr. Wilson, who fractured his skull and was unconscious for 3 weeks, survived. Upon regaining consciousness, Mr. Wilson had retrograde amnesia and was unable to recall the circumstances surrounding the incident. He was initially found incompetent to stand trial due to his retrograde amnesia, and a district court judge had him committed to St. Elizabeth's Hospital in Washington, DC, for 14 months. In November 1966, he was found competent to stand trial and convicted. On appeal, Mr. Wilson raised the question as to whether "it is a denial of due process [fair trial per the Fifth Amendment] or of the right to effective assistance of counsel [Sixth Amendment] to try a defendant suffering from such a loss of memory." The U.S. Court of Appeals, District of Columbia Circuit, found that a loss of memory does not necessarily preclude proceeding to trial, but that the trial court must consider if there is sufficient extrinsic information about what happened, whether the defendant can follow the proceedings against him, discuss the proceedings rationally with his attorney, and testify on his own behalf, and the strength of the state's case. The case was remanded for consideration of the above.

JACKSON V. INDIANA, 406 U.S. 715 (1972)

Link to case: http://scholar.google.com/scholar_case?
case=3353749416334368664

Question: Can a defendant be committed indefinitely if he is found incompetent to stand trial but not restorable?

Answer: No.

In 1968, Theon Jackson was charged in Marion, Indiana, with two counts of robbery of two women whose stolen items were valued at $9. A competency evaluation was ordered, as he was described as a "deaf mute" who was unable to read and write and who communicated only through limited sign language. He was found incompetent to stand trial, and both examiners found it unlikely that he would improve over the long term. He was committed to the Indiana Department of Mental Health until the department could certify that Mr. Jackson was "sane." Mr. Jackson's counsel filed a motion for a new trial, contending that there was no evidence that his client was "insane," nor was there evidence that he would ever be restored to competence for the purposes of standing trial. His counsel argued that the commitment amounted to a "life sentence" without a conviction and therefore deprived Mr. Jackson of his rights to due process and equal protection under the Fourteenth Amendment and violated the Eighth Amendment prohibition against cruel and unusual punishment. The trial court denied his motion, and the Supreme Court of Indiana affirmed the denial. The U.S. Supreme Court reversed and agreed with Mr. Jackson's argument. The court also stated that indefinite commitment as a result of incompetency violated due process. "Due process at least requires the nature and duration of commitment bear some reasonable relation to the purpose for which the individual is committed." Therefore, an incompetent defendant cannot be held more than what is considered a reasonable period of time to determine "whether there is a substantial probability that he will attain that capacity in the foreseeable future." If capacity restoration is unlikely, civil commitment proceedings would be required to justify further confinement.

DROPE V. MISSOURI, 420 U.S. 162 (1975)

Link to case: http://scholar.google.com/scholar_case?case=12110713099598535891

Question: Should a judge interrupt criminal proceedings if a defendant appears to be incompetent?

Answer: Yes.

In February 1969, James Drope was indicted with two other men on charges of raping his wife. His counsel filed a motion for continuance in order for Mr. Drope to be examined and receive psychiatric treatment. When this motion was initially rejected, counsel expressed that Mr. Drope was not of sound mind and requested further psychiatric evaluation before the case went to trial. His objection was denied, and the case proceeded forward. After his wife's testimony on the first day of the trial, during which she noted his bizarre behavior and an attempt to choke her on the preceding day, Mr. Drope shot himself in the abdomen. When he failed to show up to court the next morning, his counsel moved for a mistrial, which was denied. Mr. Drope was convicted and sentenced to life in prison.

Mr. Drope's counsel filed a motion for a new trial, which was denied. In 1971, Mr. Drope filed a motion to vacate his judgment and conviction, claiming that in not ordering a psychiatric examination prior to trial and conducting the trial in his absence the state had violated his constitutional rights. This motion was again denied. On appeal to the U.S. Supreme Court, the Court concluded that the record revealed a failure to give proper weight to the information that came to light at the trial suggesting Mr. Drope's incompetence. In addition, it noted that the Court should reconsider competence at any point in a trial where circumstances suggest a change that would render the accused unable to meet the standards of competency to stand trial. In Mr. Drope's case, there was sufficient evidence to question his competency, and the correct course was to suspend the trial until competency evaluation could be completed. The conviction and sentence were reversed, and the case was remanded. The Court also noted that the state was free to retry Mr. Drope, assuming that he was competent to be tried.

MEDINA V. CALIFORNIA, 505 U.S. 437 (1992)

Link: https://supreme.justia.com/cases/federal/us/505/437/

Question: Is it a violation of the Due Process Clause of the Fourteenth Amendment to place the burden of proof on the defendant to demonstrate incompetence to stand trial?

Answer: No.

Teofilo Medina, Jr., was arrested and charged with multiple offense, including three counts of first-degree murder, following a crime spree during which he killed three employees of the places he robbed. Medina's attorney requested an evaluation for competence to stand trial, under a California statute under which "it shall be presumed that the defendant is mentally competent unless it is proved by a preponderance of the evidence that the defendant is mentally incompetent." At Medina's criminal trial, the jury heard conflicting expert testimony about his mental condition. The four psychiatrists who testified disagreed about the diagnosis, as well as whether or not Medina was incompetent to stand trial.

As a result of the inconsistencies in the expert testimony, Medina argued that because psychiatry is an inexact science, a defendant may have to bear the risk of being forced to stand trial after an erroneous finding of competency, and thus placing the burden of proof on the defendant violates due process. In addressing Medina's arguments, the Supreme Court reviewed the historical treatment of the burden of proof in competency proceedings and concluded that the allocation of the burden of proof to a criminal defendant to prove incompetence "does not offend some principle of justice so rooted in the traditions and conscience of our people as to be ranked as fundamental" (quoting from *Patterson v. New York*, 432 U.S. 197, 202 (1977)). The Court found that despite the inexact science of psychiatry and differentiation of reasonable minds as to the wisdom of placing the burden of proof on the defendant in these circumstances, the State was not required to adopt one procedure over another on the basis that it may produce results more favorable to the accused. Thus, as long as a State provided a defendant access to procedures for making a competency evaluation, due process was satisfied.

GODINEZ V. MORAN, 509 U.S. 389 (1993)

Link to case: http://scholar.google.com/scholar_case?
case=13448720628873766473

Question: Is the standard to waive constitutional rights higher than the standard for competency to stand trial?

Answer: No.

Richard Moran entered the Red Pearl Saloon in Las Vegas, Nevada, on August 2, 1984, and shot and killed the bartender and a bar patron before removing the cash register. Nine days later, he shot and killed his former wife before shooting himself in the abdomen and slitting his wrists.

Mr. Moran survived, and on August 13, he confessed to the killings. After pleading not guilty to three counts of first-degree murder, he was found competent to stand trial by two psychiatrists. Mr. Moran subsequently informed the court that he wished to dismiss his attorneys and change his plea to guilty. The court accepted his waiver of counsel and his guilty pleas. A three-judge court sentenced him to death on January 21, 1985. In 1987, he sought postconviction relief in the state court on grounds that he was incompetent to represent himself, but the trial court and the Supreme Court of Nevada rejected this claim. He subsequently filed a writ of habeas corpus petition in the U.S. District Court of Nevada, which was denied. The Ninth Circuit reversed, concluding that the Due Process Clause of the Fourteenth Amendment required the court to hold a hearing with regard to Mr. Moran's competency before accepting his dismissal of counsel and change of plea. The Ninth Circuit specifically stated that competency to waive constitutional rights required a higher level of mental functioning, which it termed a "reasoned choice" standard. The U.S. Supreme Court reversed, rejecting the notion that competency in matters of pleading guilty or waiving right counsel was to be measured by a higher standard than the one outlined in *Dusky v. U.S.*

COOPER V. OKLAHOMA, 517 U.S. 348 (1996)

Link to case: http://scholar.google.com/scholar_case?
case=2215296136817695478

Question: Is preponderance of the evidence the appropriate standard for deciding a defendant is competent to stand trial?

Answer: Yes.

Mr. Cooper was charged in the murder of an 86-year-old man in 1989. A jury found him guilty of first-degree murder, and the court concurred with the jury's recommendation of the death penalty. On five separate occasions before and during the trial, Mr. Cooper's competence was called into question. His behavior over the course of the trial included refusing to change out of his prison garb because he believed the clothes were "burning" him, talking to himself and an imaginary "spirit" who provided him counsel, and expressing a fear that his counsel wanted to kill him. Mr. Cooper's attorney moved for a mistrial or additional investigation into his competence but was denied. The Court of Criminal Appeals rejected the argument that Oklahoma's presumption of competence and statutory requirement that incompetence be established by clear and convincing evidence violated his due process. The U.S. Supreme Court reversed on appeal, finding that the heightened standard of clear and convincing evidence was not protective of the defendant's rights under the Due Process Clause of the Fourteenth Amendment because it "imposes a significant risk of erroneous determination" that an incompetent defendant is found competent. The result of such a determination threatens the "basic fairness of the trial itself," and the defendant's right to be tried while competent outweighs the state's interest in operating an efficient criminal justice system. The standard of proof must be preponderance of the evidence.

INDIANA V. EDWARDS, 554 U.S. 164 (2008)

Link to case: https://scholar.google.com/scholar_case?
case=1997935653676212335&q=indiana+v+edwards&hl=en&as_sdt=6,39

Question: Can a state deny a defendant the right to self-representation, despite having been found competent to stand trial?

Answer: Yes.

Ahmad Edwards, a man with schizophrenia, attempted to steal a pair of shoes from the Parisian Department Store in Indianapolis in July 1999. After being discovered, he fired a gun at a store security guard, injuring a bystander. Mr. Edwards fled and was apprehended by an FBI agent, who shot him in the thigh after Mr. Edwards refused to drop his weapon. He was charged with attempted murder. Mr. Edwards was found incompetent to stand trial three times. After his third restoration, he asked to represent himself. This request was denied at both the first trial where he was convicted only of criminal recklessness and robbery, as well as when he was subsequently retried on the attempted murder and battery charges. The trial judge found him competent to stand trial, but not to defend himself. Mr. Edwards was convicted on the remaining charges. He appealed to the intermediate appellate court in Indiana, arguing that the refusal to permit him to represent himself denied him his constitutional right of self-representation. The court agreed and ordered a new trial. On appeal by the state, the Indiana Supreme Court affirmed the intermediate appellate court's decision, finding that Mr. Edwards's Sixth Amendment right to self-representation had been violated. The U.S. Supreme Court vacated the judgment of the Supreme Court of Indiana and remanded the case for further proceedings, stating that the standard outlined in *Dusky* applied to those with counsel, and that *Godinez* only referred to waiving of the right to counsel, not ability to act as your own counsel. The standard for competency to stand trial was not necessarily the same as the standard to determine competency for defendants to conduct trial proceedings by themselves. Therefore, the U.S. Constitution permits states to insist upon representation by counsel for those incompetent to conduct trial proceedings by themselves but competent to stand trial under *Dusky*.

TRUEBLOOD V. WASHINGTON STATE DEPARTMENT OF SOCIAL AND HEALTH SERVICES, 822 F.3D 1037 (2016)

Link to case: https://caselaw.findlaw.com/us-9th-circuit/1734234.html

Question: Does prolonged wait time while incarcerated for competency evaluation and/or restoration services constitute a violation of the Due Process Clause of the Fourteenth Amendment?

Answer: Yes.

Trueblood was a class action lawsuit that enforced a person's constitutional right to a timely competency evaluation and restoration services. The class members consisted of persons who were waiting in jail for court-ordered competency evaluations and restoration services. Washington state law charged the Washington State Department of Social and Health Services (DSHS) with overseeing the competency evaluations and restoration services and set a target deadline of seven days for DSHS to complete such competency evaluations and restoration services for individuals in jails. The class action suit alleged that the consistent failure to meet the target deadlines resulted in the confinement of individuals in county and city jails for weeks and months without appropriate mental health treatment, in violation of the Due Process Clause of the Fourteenth Amendment.

The district court found in favor of the plaintiffs and issued an injunction to prevent the incarceration of persons for more than 7 days while they waited for DSHS to provide competency services, without an individualized determination by a court of good cause to continue incarceration of that person. The district court reasoned that the gravity of the harms suffered by class members during prolonged incarceration (including increased instances of solitary confinement, mental health deterioration, victimization, and longer restoration time due to symptom chronicity) directly conflicted with rights to freedom from incarceration and to the competency services which form the basis of their detention. The court also opined that the prolonged incarceration directly conflicted with the State's speedy trial interests and adjudication process.

The United States Court of Appeals for the Ninth Circuit agreed with the district court that DSHS must conduct competency evaluations within a reasonable time following a court's order, but that the 7-day mandate imposed a temporal obligation beyond what the Constitution required, and so the case was remanded back to the district court to amend the injunction. In 2018, a settlement agreement was reached. The agreement required the State to make changes in five substantive areas: competency evaluations; competency restoration services; crisis triage and diversion support; education and training; and workforce development.

CHAPTER 23

ⳙ

Diminished Capacity

MICHAEL GREENSPAN

PEOPLE V. PATTERSON, 39 N.Y.2D 288 (1976)

Link to case: http://scholar.google.com/scholar_case?
case=6754859816004446983

Question: Is it constitutional in New York to place the burden of proof for
extreme emotional disturbance (EED) on the defendant?

Answer: Yes.

Gordon Patterson had an unstable and abusive relationship with his wife.
In December 1970, Mr. Patterson observed his wife scantily dressed with
John Northrup, her paramour. Mr. Patterson shot Mr. Northrup twice in
the head at close range. At trial, Mr. Patterson claimed both that the gun
had gone off accidentally and that he had been acting in a state of extreme
emotional disturbance. Under the New York statute, EED could potentially
mitigate a murder conviction to manslaughter. The burden of proving EED
was placed on the defendant. At trial, Mr. Patterson was found guilty of
murder. He unsuccessfully appealed, based on the primary contention that
his due process right under the Fourteenth Amendment had been violated
because the jury had been instructed that the defense bore the burden to
prove EED. The New York Court of Appeals affirmed the decision against Mr.
Patterson, holding that the New York EED law did not negate the "fundamental" constitutional principle that the state must prove all the elements
of a crime. As opposed to the unconstitutional Maine statute upon which
Patterson based his appeal in which the emotional disturbance negated intent, in New York EED does not negate the intent that the prosecution

must prove, so placing the burden of proving EED on the defense does not violate due process.

IBN-TAMAS V. U.S. 407 A.2D 626 (1979)

Link to case: http://scholar.google.com/scholar_case?
case=8618054616035755185

Question: Should testimony about a recognized syndrome in a defendant be excluded from evidence because of its potential prejudicial impact on the jury?

Answer: No.

Beverly Ibn-Tamas was convicted of second-degree murder in the Superior Court of Washington, DC. Ms. Ibn-Tamas had shot her husband after years of physical abuse at his hands. On the morning of the incident, her husband had assaulted her, pointed a gun at her head, and told her to leave the family's residence or suffer severe retribution. At trial, the defense attempted to enter testimony of Dr. Lenore Walker, a clinical psychologist. Dr. Walker discussed the "battered woman syndrome." She opined that the defendant did, in fact, suffer from said syndrome and therefore was acting in what in her mind was self-defense. The trial court did not allow entry of this evidence, feeling that it would infringe on the province of the jury to assess the credibility of witnesses and that it presupposed that her husband was, in fact, a batterer. The DC Court of Appeals reversed the decision, stating that the testimony should not have been excluded. It reasoned that the expert was providing important background information that was "beyond the ken" of an ordinary jury. Therefore, the probative value of the information outweighed any potential prejudicial effect. The court further found that the record did not clearly establish that the record did not establish that the methodology underpinning Dr. Walker's fell short of the necessary general acceptance required for the admissibility of scientific expertise. The case was remanded for further consideration, including the now admissible testimony.

PEOPLE V. SAILLE, 820 P.2D 588 (1991)

Link to case: http://scholar.google.com/scholar_case?
case=10687954333870937195

Issue: Can voluntary intoxication be used to reduce a murder charge to manslaughter in California?

Answer: No.

Manuel De Jesus Saille became severely drunk at a local bar, Eva's Café, in California. Upon being "turned down" twice for more alcohol, Mr. Saille left the bar after threatening to return and kill the bartender. He returned with a firearm. In the struggle that ensued with the bar's security, a by-stander was shot and killed. Mr. Saille's blood alcohol level several hours after the shooting was 0.14. Mr. Saille was found guilty of murder at trial and appealed based on the contention that the jury instruction that voluntary intoxication was only relevant to "specific intent to kill" was inadequate. The court of appeals, and ultimately the California Supreme Court, affirmed the trial court's guilty finding. The court opined that the state's new penal law had limited voluntary intoxication as a defense to cases only where there was evidence that, as a result, the defendant actually did not form the required specific intent, and not merely that his capacity to form the intent was impaired. The required specific intent in this murder case was a premeditated decision to kill another person. Voluntary intoxication, alone, could not be a reason for reducing the crime to manslaughter.

MONTANA V. EGELHOFF, 518 U.S. 37 (1996)

Link to case: http://scholar.google.com/scholar_case?
case=2969282020576743127

Question: Does the Montana law excluding evidence about voluntary intoxication as related to mental state in a criminal offense violate due process?

Answer: No.

In July 1992, James Egelhoff met Roberta Pavola and John Christenson while camping in Montana. The group picked mushrooms and soon engaged in a night of binge drinking. At around midnight, police officers discovered Mr. Egelhoff in the back of the car, shouting obscenities and with a blood alcohol level of 0.36. Ms. Pavola and Mr. Christenson lay dead in the car, each with a single gunshot wound to the head. Mr. Egelhoff had gun residue on his hands, and the weapon of the crime lay on the floor of the parked car. The Montana statute of murder required that the defendant "purposely" or "knowingly" engaged in the murderous act. In accordance with Montana criminal law, the trial jury was instructed not to consider the defendant's drunkenness at the time of the crime and ultimately found Egelhoff guilty. The Montana Supreme Court reversed the guilty finding, reasoning that the due process protections under the Fourteenth Amendment require that all relevant evidence, including that of voluntary intoxication, be considered. On certiorari, the U.S. Supreme Court reversed the appeal, agreeing with the trial court's suppression of this mental state evidence. The Court relied on historical and common law arguments to hold that the exclusion of voluntary intoxication in violent crimes was not a violation of due process.

CHAPTER 24

⁂

Insanity

KATYA FRISCHER

M'NAGHTEN'S CASE, 8 ENG. REP. 718 (1843)

Link to case: http://www.bailii.org/uk/cases/UKHL/1843/J16.html

Question: Can a defendant be found not guilty by reason of insanity (NGRI) in a criminal case if, as a result of mental illness, he cognitively did not know what he was doing or that it was wrong?

Answer: Yes.

On January 20, 1843, Mr. M'Naghten shot British prime minister Robert Peel's secretary, Mr. Drummond, while attempting to shoot Mr. Peel. Mr. Drummond died from his wounds. M'Naghten was found NGRI by the jury. Evidence presented in court indicated Mr. M'Naghten was mentally ill with persecutory delusions, which resulted in his inability to control his behavior at the time of the crime. Due to public outrage, Queen Victoria appealed to the judges in the House of Lords to answer general questions about the standard for legal insanity (e.g., What is the law regarding a defendant's guilt if he is afflicted with delusions but knows he is acting contrary to the law? Can a physician testify as to the state of mind of a defendant if he did not examine him prior to trial?). The judges opined that in order to be adjudicated not guilty by reason of insanity the defendant had to be mentally ill to the extent that he did not know what he was doing or, if he knew what he is doing, that he did not know that what he was doing was wrong. This cognitive, knowledge of right-and-wrong criterion has come to be known as the M'Naghten standard.

DURHAM V. U.S. 214 F.2D 862 (1954)

Link to case: http://scholar.google.com/scholar_case?
case=1244686235948852364

Question: Is the *M'Naghten* "right/wrong" standard for legal insanity, even when modified to include irresistible impulse, too narrow? Should a more "modern" criterion reflect whether or not the defendant's criminal act was the product of a mental disease or defect?

Answer: Yes.

In 1954, the U.S. Court of Appeals, District of Columbia Circuit, reviewed the trial court's conviction of Monte Durham for burglary. Mr. Durham had a well-documented history of mental illness since the age of 17. He was reported to have suffered hallucinations and had been hospitalized several times at St. Elizabeth's Psychiatric Hospital. He had been variably diagnosed with "psychosis with psychopathic personality" as well as "without mental disorder, psychopathic personality." The Court of Appeals reversed Mr. Durham's conviction on two grounds: (1) the trial court erred in stating that there was "no" evidence of mental disorder, when there was "some" evidence; this evidence was sufficient to overcome the presumption of sanity and should have shifted the burden to the state to prove sanity, and (2) more modern conceptions of the integration of cognitive and behavioral mental processes and potential confusion about the necessity for sudden onset in assessing impulsivity mean that the standard for legal insanity should be changed to "product of mental disease or defect" from the existing *M'Naghten* right/wrong and/or irresistible impulse test. This was known as the *Durham*, or product, rule.

WASHINGTON V. U.S., 390 F.2D 444 (1967)

Link to case: http://scholar.google.com/scholar_case?
case=11121900497855531360

Question: Should an expert witness be allowed to testify to the ultimate question in an insanity defense case?

Answer: No.

Thomas Washington was convicted by jury of rape, robbery, and assault with a deadly weapon in Washington, D.C., following an unsuccessful insanity defense. Mr. Washington appealed the conviction to the U.S. Court of Appeals for the D.C. Circuit. The court found that the psychiatric evidence presented at trial was "more confusing than clarifying," at times omitted important evidence, and was an "abstract mass of philosophical discussion." However, it reasoned that although much of the information presented to the jury may not have been dispositive, full of medical jargon, and confusing, the jury ultimately got enough facts to be able to make a decision regarding the defendant's mental illness and culpability. The court, in an opinion by Justice David Bazelon, ruled that the jury, not the psychiatric experts, should decide to what extent the alleged offense was a *product* of mental illness. The court advised that the trial judge should give explanatory instructions in open court regarding the proper role of the expert and the jury.

FRENDAK V. U.S., 408 A.2D 364 (1979)

Link to case: http://scholar.google.com/scholar_case?
case=8884757738165900061

Question: Can a defendant with mental illness whose sanity at the time of the crime is in question competently refuse to raise an insanity defense?

Answer: Yes.

Paula Frendak was convicted of first-degree homicide in Washington, D.C., in 1974, for killing a coworker, Willard Titlow, and carrying a pistol without a license. After the shooting, Ms. Frendak left Washington and traveled abroad until she was extradited to Washington from Abu Dhabi. She had a history of mental illness, including a history of hallucinations and delusions. She had several competency hearings and was found competent to stand trial on the fourth evaluation. After her conviction, she appealed, stating that the trial judge inappropriately raised the insanity defense over her competent objections. While an earlier appellate court decision (*Whalem v. United States*, 346 F.2d 8120) allowed for the imposition of the insanity defense, Frendak argued the subsequent Supreme Court decisions (*North Carolina v. Alford*, 400 U.S. 25 and *Faretta v. California*, 422 U.S. 806) which supported the rights of a defendant to control her own defense should allow a defendant to refuse to plead insanity. The D.C. Court of Appeals agreed. The court enumerated several good reasons to decline an insanity defense, including avoidance of indefinite confinement, objection to mental health treatment, concern about stigma, loss of other rights, and the desire to make a political statement. The court ruled that if a defendant has acted intelligently and voluntarily, a trial court must defer to his or her decision to waive the insanity defense. However, the trial court should have the ability to raise the defense if a defendant is not capable of making or has not made an intelligent and voluntary decision. A finding of competency to stand trial is not in and of itself a test of intelligence and voluntariness; the case was remanded to clarify if the defendant was capable of intelligently refusing the insanity defense.

JONES V. U.S., 463 U.S. 354 (1983)

Link to case: http://scholar.google.com/scholar_case?case=5221664652529148549

Question: Must a defendant found NGRI remain mentally ill and dangerous at the time of commitment and afforded the same due process delineated in *Addington vs. Texas*? Must the duration of confinement relate to the nature of the commitment offense?

Answer: No.

Michael Jones was arrested for attempting to steal a jacket from a department store in the District of Columbia. He was charged with misdemeanor petty larceny and eventually found not guilty by reason of insanity. He was committed at St. Elizabeth's Hospital with a diagnosis of schizophrenia. At a court hearing, he requested to be released or recommitted under a civil commitment statute, stating that he had been hospitalized for longer than the period he would have spent in prison if he had been convicted. He was denied and appealed to the D.C. Court of Appeals on the grounds that his Fourteenth Amendment right to due process and equal protection had been violated. The appellate court, after several hearings, affirmed the trial court finding. The U.S. Supreme Court heard the case and ruled that a finding of insanity at trial is sufficient to justify commitment at a preponderance of the evidence standard (lower than the civil commitment clear and convincing requirement), since the verdict was based on a finding of mental illness and a criminal act, which is, by definition, dangerousness. Furthermore, commitment as an insanity acquittee serves a different purpose than incarceration, and there is no necessary correlation between the severity of the offense and the length of time necessary for recovery. Insanity acquittees constitute a special class and can be treated differently from civil patients.

U.S. V. TORNIERO, 735 F.2D 725 (2D CIR. CONN. 1984)

Link to case: http://scholar.google.com/scholar_case?case=11490969042080455149

Question: Is an individual with compulsive gambling necessarily legally insane with respect to all behaviors that may be associated with his gambling behavior?

Answer: No.

John Torniero, a jewelry store manager, was indicted for interstate transportation of jewelry worth $750,000 stolen from his employer. He argued that a compulsion to gamble rendered him legally insane. After extensive testimony by psychiatrists, the trial court ruled that the relationship between gambling and the urge to steal is tenuous and was irrelevant to the issue of insanity. Mr. Torniero was convicted and then appealed to the U.S. Court of Appeals for the Second Circuit, stating that the trial judge erred by refusing to present the evidence about compulsive gambling to the jury. The court of appeals affirmed, explaining that under the American Law Institute (ALI) test a person is not responsible for criminal conduct if at the time of such conduct as a result of mental disease or defect he lacks substantial capacity either to appreciate the wrongfulness of his conduct or to conform his conduct to the requirements of the law. In this case the evidence would be relevant if the defendant could prove that compulsive gambling is a mental disease or defect capable of making him unable to resist the urge to steal. The court reasoned that in order for it to consider psychiatric evidence for the purposes of insanity, there should be substantial acceptance in the discipline that compulsive gambling is a mental illness and that there is a nexus between gambling and stealing. It found that the trial court did not abuse its discretion in determining that the proposed evidence about compulsive gambling was irrelevant.

FOUCHA V. LOUISIANA, 504 U.S. 71 (1992)

Link to case: http://scholar.google.com/scholar_case?case=15775785182348520983

Question: Must an insanity acquittee be both mentally ill and dangerous for a state to justify continued hospitalization?

Answer: Yes.

Mr. Foucha was committed to a Louisiana psychiatric hospital as an insanity acquittee. Under Louisiana law, after the hospital committee recommends that the acquittee be released, the trial court must hold a hearing to determine whether the acquittee is a danger to himself or others. The statute allowed the acquittee to be returned to the hospital for further treatment simply on the basis of dangerousness. Mr. Foucha was retained in the hospital after a psychiatrist testified at his hearing that although Mr. Foucha was not mentally ill, he continued to exhibit symptoms of antisocial personality disorder that rendered him dangerous. On appeal, the Louisiana Supreme Court confirmed the judgment; Mr. Foucha appealed. The U.S. Supreme Court reversed, reasoning that because Mr. Foucha was no longer mentally ill, it would be a violation of his due process right (as interpreted by earlier case law) to continue to hold him as a mentally ill person. The Court also found that the statute violated the Equal Protection Clause. Although, in *Jones* (see earlier) the Court held that insanity acquittees constituted their own special class for constitutional purposes, once the acquittee was no longer mentally ill, that class distinction no longer applied. In allowing continued confinement, the statute discriminated against insanity acquittees who would be retained although they do not differ from other criminals (i.e., without mental illness) who may be dangerous but whose confinement would be subject to the rules of temporary pretrial detention and the expectation of definite release at the end of their sentence.

CLARK V. ARIZONA, 548 U.S. 735 (2006)

Link to case: http://caselaw.lp.findlaw.com/scripts/getcase.pl?navby=case&court=us&vol=548&page=735

Question: Can a state restrict evidence of mental illness at the time of a crime from being used as a *mens rea* defense (as opposed to legal insanity)?

Answer: Yes.

Question: May states with insanity defense statutes constitutionally restrict the cognitive prong of legal insanity to an appreciation of wrongfulness?

Answer: Yes.

Eric Michael Clark shot and killed a police officer in Flagstaff, Arizona, and then argued at trial that he had a history of schizophrenia that included delusions that the police officer was an alien who was trying to kill him. He argued that he was therefore not guilty of the statutorily defined crime of intent to kill a police officer, and that he was also legally insane. The judge, in accordance with the Arizona penal code, denied Mr. Clark's attempt to plead lack of intent and restricted his mental illness defense to legal insanity. Mr. Clark sought to vacate the judgment based on the argument that the Arizona statute was unconstitutional because it only included the knowledge of right and wrong criterion of the M'Naghten standard (leaving out the understanding of the nature and quality of the act). Mr. Clark also argued that the judge violated his due process rights when he applied an Arizona case (also known as the "Mott rule") that did not allow evidence of mental illness for the purposes of insanity to be used to rebut evidence of criminal intent. The trial court denied Mr. Clark's request to vacate, the Arizona Court of Appeals agreed, and the U.S. Supreme Court affirmed. The Court held that that there is no constitutional right to any particular definition of legal insanity. The Court noted that not all states have an insanity defense and those that do have varying standards for legal insanity. With reference to the "Mott rule," the Court reasoned that given the potential for jury confusion when assessing expert testimony about mental illness, Arizona made a reasonable decision to confine the consideration of evidence of mental disease and incapacity to the insanity defense so that it can preserve a legal presumption of sanity and the requirement that a defendant prove his insanity.

CHAPTER 25

✢

Prisoners' Rights

OMAR KHAN, REBECCA LEWIS, BIPIN SUBEDI,
AND HEATHER ELLIS CUCOLO

ESTELLE V. GAMBLE, 429 U.S. 97 (1976)

Link to case: http://scholar.google.com/scholar_case?
case=4755107314332030951

Question: Do prisoners have a constitutional right to treatment?

Answer: Yes.

J. W. Gamble was a Texas Department of Corrections (DOC) inmate who
was injured when a bale of cotton fell on him while he was unloading
a truck. He was diagnosed with "lower back strain." Mr. Gamble was
evaluated 17 times for back pain and cardiac problems over the next
3 months. He was excused from work duties, but prison staff did not
follow through with other medical orders. He received medication with
little benefit. After several months, Mr. Gamble was medically cleared, but
he refused to go to work due to ongoing pain. He was placed in administrative segregation, then solitary confinement. Mr. Gamble sued W. J.
Estelle, director of the DOC, and other staff members, stating that their
"refusal" to provide care violated his Eighth Amendment right against
cruel and unusual punishment. The district court dismissed the com-
plaint, the U.S. Court of Appeals for the Fifth Circuit reversed/remanded,
and the U.S. Supreme Court agreed to hear the case. The Court ruled that
the Eighth Amendment, as defined by "contemporary standards of decency," supports a right to adequate medical care for prisoners, whose loss
of liberty prevents their seeking medical care on their own. However, the

Court further defined the standard for such a constitutional violation as "deliberate indifference" to a prisoner's serious medical needs, that is, intentionally denying/delaying access to medical care, not mere negligence. Mr. Gamble's care may have been negligent, but it was not necessarily deliberately indifferent. The case was remanded with instructions to apply the above standard to the others named in the suit.

VITEK V. JONES, 445 U.S. 480 (1980)

Link to case: http://scholar.google.com/scholar_case?case=12392576224835810750

Question: Is a prisoner constitutionally entitled to procedural protections before involuntary transfer to a psychiatric hospital for treatment?

Answer: Yes.

In May 1974, Larry Jones was convicted of robbery and sentenced to 3 to 9 years in the Nebraska state penitentiary. He was transferred to the penitentiary hospital in January 1975, 2 days after which he set fire to his mattress, severely burned himself, and required treatment for the burns at a private hospital. After receiving treatment for the burns, Mr. Jones was transferred to Lincoln Regional Center (a state psychiatric hospital) in accordance with Nebraska law requiring a designated physician or psychologist to find that Mr. Jones suffered from a "mental disease or defect" and could not "be given proper treatment" within the correctional institution. Mr. Jones challenged the constitutionality of this statute; the district court agreed and declared the transfer unconstitutional. The U.S. District Court opined that the transfer infringed on Mr. Jones's liberty interest protected by the Due Process Clause of the Fourteenth Amendment, including the "stigmatizing" consequences of psychiatric hospitalization and the potential imposition of involuntary treatment. In March 1980, the U.S. Supreme Court affirmed the district court decision requiring the state to abide by the following procedures before transfer of a prisoner to a mental hospital: written notice to the prisoner, a hearing allowing for presentation of evidence and testimony, an independent decision maker, a written statement by the fact finder, and legal counsel for the prisoner.

WASHINGTON V. HARPER, 494 U.S. 210 (1990)

Link to case: http://scholar.google.com/scholar_case?case=13274222040240404814

Question: Is a judicial hearing about medication required to satisfy due process for a dangerous, convicted prisoner refusing psychiatric medication?

Answer: No.

Walter Harper was incarcerated in the Washington state penal system. On two occasions, he was transferred to the Special Offender Center (SOC), a state institute for convicted felons with serious mental illness. While there, he was required to take antipsychotic medications against his will pursuant to an SOC policy, which provided that, among other due process protections, a hospital committee review the need for involuntary medication. Mr. Harper filed suit, claiming that the lack of a judicial hearing about involuntary medication violated his liberty interests under the Fourteenth Amendment. The trial court rejected his claim. The Washington State Supreme Court reversed and remanded, concluding that a judicial hearing was necessary. The U.S. Supreme Court granted certiorari. The Court ruled that Harper had a protected liberty interest in avoiding unwanted antipsychotic medication. However, the Court held that this liberty interest must be balanced against the state interest in "prison safety and security." It noted the following: (1) there is a legitimate state interest in combating danger posed by a violent mentally ill inmate, and (2) there is little dispute that proper use of medications is an effective means of treating mental illness. The Court held that the SOC policy satisfied both substantive and procedural due process and reversed the Washington State Supreme Court ruling. In addition, the Court wrote that liberty interests might be better served by allowing medical professionals rather than a judge to make the decision to medicate. The SOC policy fulfilled procedural due process by mandating notice of a hearing, the right to representation by a disinterested adviser, and the right to appeal to the state court.

RIGGINS V. NEVADA, 504 U.S. 127 (1992)

Link to case: http://scholar.google.com/scholar_case?case=7905994277524677132

Question: Can a person standing trial be forced to take antipsychotic medication without a determination that it is both medically appropriate and the least intrusive option?

Answer: No.

David Riggins was charged with murder. He was prescribed thioridazine for auditory hallucinations and was found competent to stand trial. The defense moved to suspend thioridazine during the trial, arguing that the medication's effects on Mr. Riggins's demeanor would affect the jury's opinion of him and, therefore, deny him a fair trial. The district court denied the motion. Mr. Riggins presented an insanity defense and was convicted and sentenced to death. He appealed, arguing that the forced administration of thioridazine violated his right to assist in his defense, and, that the state should have demonstrated treatment with antipsychotics over objection was medically necessary and least restrictive. The Nevada Supreme Court affirmed his conviction and death sentence. The U.S. Supreme Court granted certiorari and reversed the decision. Referring to *Washington v. Harper*, the Court found that forcing antipsychotic medications on a convicted prisoner is impermissible without overriding compelling state interest and a determination of medical appropriateness. The Court found that the Fourteenth Amendment affords at least as much protection to persons standing trial as to those convicted and sentenced. The Court found that the lower court decisions neither explicitly affirmed this liberty interest, nor did they indicate a finding of a safety or other compelling state interest that could override the liberty interest. Therefore, the Court remanded the case for further consideration and did not directly address whether a person may be medicated forcibly for the purpose of maintaining competence to stand trial.

FARMER V. BRENNAN, 511 U.S. 825 (1994)

Link to case: http://scholar.google.com/scholar_case?case=2417836767044325448

Question: Does the "deliberate indifference" standard outlined in *Estelle v. Gamble* require actual knowledge of risk by prison officials?

Answer: Yes.

Dee Farmer, a male-to-female preoperative transsexual, was convicted of credit card fraud and sentenced to federal prison in 1986. In 1989, Ms. Farmer was transferred to a higher-security facility for disciplinary reasons. Following this transfer, Ms. Farmer was allegedly beaten and raped by a male inmate in her cell. Ms. Farmer filed a civil suit alleging an Eighth Amendment violation against prison officials for being deliberately indifferent with regard to protecting her safety. The U.S. District Court granted summary judgment to the prison officials that was affirmed by the U.S. Court of Appeals for the Seventh Circuit. The U.S. Supreme Court heard the case and decided that prison officials may be held liable for deliberate indifference only if they are aware of a "substantial risk of serious harm" and they "disregard that risk by failing to take reasonable measures to abate it." According to the ruling, deliberate indifference is somewhere above negligence but below purposeful or knowledgeable harm, and the appropriate test for this case was determined to be that of subjective recklessness: "The official must both be aware of facts from which the inference could be drawn that a substantial risk of serious harm exists, *and he must also draw the inference* (emphasis added). The U.S. Supreme Court vacated the decision and remanded the case for further review.

SELL V. U.S., 539 U.S. 166 (2003)

Link to case: http://scholar.google.com/scholar_case?
case=10071406451224631321

Question: Can antipsychotic drugs be forced on a defendant facing serious criminal charges in order to restore competence to stand trial?

Answer: Yes.

Charles Sell was a dentist with a psychotic disorder who was indicted for health care fraud and attempted murder in Missouri. Dr. Sell was found incompetent to stand trial and, while hospitalized, refused antipsychotic medication. The magistrate authorized forced administration of antipsychotic medication, finding that Dr. Sell was dangerous. The district court found the magistrate's dangerousness finding erroneous but concluded that medication was necessary to render Dr. Sell competent to stand trial and, therefore, necessary to serve the government interest in adjudicating his case. The U.S. Court of Appeals for the Eighth Circuit affirmed, finding that the government had an essential interest in bringing Dr. Sell to trial and that the treatment was medically appropriate. The U.S. Supreme Court granted certiorari and found that the Constitution permits the government to administer antipsychotic medications involuntarily to mentally ill defendants in order to restore competence to stand trial if (1) "important government interests are at stake" (i.e., the crime is a serious one against person or property), (2) the treatment is medically appropriate, (3) the treatment is in fact likely to "render the defendant competent," (4) the treatment is "substantially unlikely to have side effects that will interfere significantly with the defendant's ability to assist counsel," and (5) taking account of less intrusive alternatives, the treatment is necessary to further governmental trial-related interests. The Court noted that in some cases forced medication under a police power or *parens patriae* justification might obviate the need for a determination of the need to decide the medication for restoration question, and it appeared to prefer that path if available. Because the original decisions reviewed by the lower federal courts were based only on Sell's dangerousness, the Court concluded that there was insufficient evidence to apply the necessary constitutional criteria it established. Consequently, the case was remanded for further consideration.

BROWN V. PLATA, 563 U.S. 493 (2011)

Link to case: http://scholar.google.com/scholar_case?
case=4913884626785841743

Question: Was a special district court ruling to drastically reduce the inmate population in California's prison system necessary and authorized by Congress?

Answer: Yes.

Brown v. Plata is a consolidation of two class action cases brought against the governor of California (Brown) alleging violations of Eighth Amendment rights in the California prison system. *Coleman v. Brown*, filed in 1990, involves a class of prisoners with serious mental disorders, and *Plata v. Brown*, filed in 2001, involves a class of prisoners with serious medical conditions. In 2008, after years of failures of remedial plans related to both cases and conditions that did not meet the minimally adequate standard, and, in accordance with the Prison Litigation Reform Act (PLRA) of 1995, a three-judge district court was convened to assess whether overcrowding was the source of the constitutional violations. If so, according to the PLRA, the court needed to find by clear and convincing evidence that there was no appropriate remedy other than reducing the prison population and that such a remedy must be narrowly tailored and issued only after strong consideration of the impact on public safety. The court determined that for more than a decade the California prison system had been operating at almost double the capacity that it was designed to accommodate. As a result, the system was unable to meet the basic health care needs of its inmates. The court ordered that the prison population be reduced to 137.5% of its designed capacity within 2 years. The State of California appealed the decision, but the U.S. Supreme Court affirmed, finding that the district court was convened appropriately, and that overcrowding was the primary cause of the substandard prison health care conditions.

TAYLOR V. BARKES, 135 S. CT. 2042 (2015)

Link to case: https://www.leagle.com/decision/insco20150601c54

Question: Does the lack of adequate suicide prevention protocols violate a prisoner's Eighth Amendment constitutional right to be free from cruel and unusual punishment?

Answer: No.

Christopher Barkes was arrested for violating his probation and was taken to the Howard R. Young Correctional Institution in Wilmington, Delaware. At intake, Barkes was administered a mental health screening designed in part to assess whether he was suicidal. Barkes had an extensive history of mental health problems and prior suicide attempts, but during the intake, he verbally affirmed that he was not currently thinking of harming himself. A suicidal screening form, consisting of seventeen suicide factors, identified only two risk factors for Barkes. After the evaluation, he was placed in a cell by himself and referred to "routine" mental health services without any initiation of special suicide prevention measures. Later that evening, Barkes called his wife to say that he could no "longer live this way." Barkes's wife did not inform the institution about the statements made during their call. The following morning, correctional officers observed Barkes acting normally, but at lunchtime, officers discovered that he had hanged himself with a sheet in his cell.

Barkes's wife and children sued Stanley Taylor, commissioner of the Delaware Department of Correction, and Raphael Williams, the warden of the institution under Rev. Stat. § 1979, 42 U.S.C. § 1983. The suit alleged that Barkes's constitutional right to be free from cruel and unusual punishment was violated by the failure of the institution to supervise and monitor the private contractor that provided the medical treatment, including the intake screening. The defendant's motion for summary judgment, based on the argument that they were entitled to qualified immunity because they did not violate a clearly established constitutional right, was denied by the district court. The U.S. Court of Appeals for the Third Circuit affirmed the denial of summary judgment.

The Supreme Court reversed the judgment of the Third Circuit. The Court held that there was no violation of a clearly established law that gave incarcerated persons the right to adequate suicide prevention protocols under the Eighth Amendment. The Court concluded its opinion by surmising that even if the institution's suicide screening and prevention measures were deficient, there was no precedent on the books at the time of Barkes's intake and confinement that would have made it clear to the administrators of the institution that they were overseeing a system that violated the Constitution. Thus, because defendants did not contravene a clearly established law, they were entitled to qualified immunity.

CHAPTER 26

Death Penalty

TARA STRAKA, HEATHER ELLIS CUCOLO,
MERRILL ROTTER, AND JEREMY COLLEY

ESTELLE V. SMITH, 451 U.S. 454 (1981)

Link to case: http://scholar.google.com/scholar_case?
case=3874052948546256691

Question: Is information gathered as part of a pretrial psychiatric evaluation admissible during the sentencing phase of a death penalty case, when
used for that purpose without the knowledge or consent of the defendant
at the time of the evaluation?

Answer: No.

Ernest Smith sought habeas corpus relief after receiving a death sentence
for murder. Mr. Smith challenged the way psychiatric evidence about him
had been obtained and used against him at sentencing. When Mr. Smith
was indicted for murder and Texas announced its intention to seek the
death penalty, the trial court ordered a psychiatric examination for competency to stand trial. Dr. James Grigson evaluated Mr. Smith without
defense counsel's awareness and found him fit to proceed. Mr. Smith was
tried by a jury and convicted. During the penalty phase, Dr. Grigson was
called as a prosecution witness and testified about Mr. Smith's potential for
future dangerousness based on his pretrial examination. The U.S. Court of
Appeals, Fifth Circuit found that Mr. Smith's protection from self-incrimination (Fifth Amendment) and his right to counsel (Sixth Amendment)
had been violated. The U.S. Supreme Court agreed. The Court noted that
the prosecution used Mr. Smith's "own statement, unwittingly made

without an awareness that he was assisting the State's efforts to obtain the death penalty."

AKE V. OKLAHOMA, 470 U.S. 68 (1985)

Link to case: http://scholar.google.com/scholar_case?
case=1904002630366313299

Question: Does the state have to provide access to a psychiatric evaluation for an indigent defendant in a case where legal insanity is at issue?

Answer: Yes.

Glen Ake was arrested for murder. At arraignment, his behavior was so bizarre that the judge ordered a competency evaluation. He was found incompetent to stand trial and was committed to the state psychiatric hospital for restoration. Mr. Ake subsequently pled insanity and requested that a psychiatrist be appointed at state expense to evaluate his state of mind at the time of the offense. The judge denied the request, and the defense called the treating psychiatrists from the state hospital. However, none of them could testify to Mr. Ake's mental state at the time of the offense because they had not evaluated such during his treatment. He was found guilty and sentenced to death, which was upheld on appeal. The U.S. Supreme Court found that it is a violation of the Fourteenth Amendment's guarantee of due process for the state to deny the defendant a psychiatric consultant "who will conduct an appropriate examination and assist in evaluation, preparation, and presentation of the defense." The Court remanded the case for a new trial. However, the Court also ruled that the defense was not necessarily entitled to a consultant of his choosing.

FORD V. WAINWRIGHT, 477 U.S. 399 (1986)

Link to case: http://scholar.google.com/scholar_case?
case=7904262174469084060

Question: Can an insane prisoner be executed?

Answer: No.

In 1974, Alvin Ford was convicted of murdering a police officer and sentenced to death. He became delusional after sentencing. Two psychiatrists hired by the defense found him incompetent to be executed, but three psychiatrists appointed by the governor found him competent based on a 30-minute interview. No adversarial hearing or cross-examination of any psychiatrist was permitted, and the governor did not acknowledge reports submitted by the defense counsel. Without explanation, the governor signed the death warrant. Mr. Ford filed a habeas corpus petition alleging that the procedures under which his competency to be executed was upheld were unconstitutional. After the 11th Circuit Court of Appeals affirmed the sentence, Mr. Ford appealed to the U.S. Supreme Court. The Court found the Florida statute governing this competency determination was unconstitutional because it allowed the finding to be carried out by the executive branch. The Court opined that a "full and fair hearing" was required, noting that this level of due process was required because execution of the insane is inherently offensive and does not meet the goals of either retribution or deterrence. In his concurring opinion, Justice Powell laid out what has become the generally accepted standard of competence to be executed: "that the Eighth Amendment forbids the execution only of those who are unaware of the punishment they are about to suffer and why they are to suffer it."

PAYNE V. TENNESSEE, 501 U.S. 808 (1991)

Link to case: http://scholar.google.com/scholar_case?case=7795411704028596196

Question: Is the inclusion of victim impact statements during the sentencing phase of a capital trial a violation of the Eighth Amendment?

Answer: No.

Pervis Tyrone Payne was convicted of capital murder after a brutal attack on a family in which he murdered a mother and her 2-year-old daughter and severely wounded her 3-year-old son. At sentencing, the 3-year-old victim's grandmother testified for the state about how the boy was affected by the crime and the loss of his mother and sister. Mr. Payne appealed his death sentence, claiming that his Eighth Amendment rights had been violated by the state's presentation of the grandmother's testimony. The state supreme court ruled that victim impact evidence can be presented; the U.S. Supreme Court affirmed. The U.S. Supreme Court had previously ruled in *Booth v. Maryland* and *South Carolina v. Gathers* that such evidence could not be presented at a capital trial sentencing phase. However, the Court now noted that *stare decisis* is not an "inexorable command," and "when governing decisions are unworkable or are badly reasoned, 'this Court has never felt constrained to follow precedent.'" It reasoned that the prior decision "unfairly weighted the scales in a capital trial" by preventing the state from countering mitigating evidence presented by the defense. It noted that victim impact statements show the specific harm caused by the crime, which aids the jury in assessing the defendant's moral culpability and also shows the victim as a unique individual.

STATE V. PERRY, 610 SO. 2D 746 (LA. 1992)

Link to case: http://scholar.google.com/scholar_case?
case=12731842654315565192

Question: Can a state involuntarily treat a death row prisoner with antipsychotic drugs to make him competent to be executed?

Answer: No.

Michael Owen Perry, a man with a long history of mental illness and a diagnosis of schizophrenia, was convicted and sentenced to death for murdering his parents, two cousins, and a nephew. His conviction was affirmed on appeal; however, the court ordered an evaluation of his competence to be executed. The trial court found him competent and ordered that he continue treatment with haloperidol to maintain his competence—even if that meant treating him over his objection. Mr. Perry appealed, but the U.S. Supreme Court sent the case back to the state for consideration pursuant to the standards it set under *Washington v. Harper*, that is, the balancing of an inmate's liberty interests in avoiding unwanted treatment, his medical need for that treatment, and the state's interest in prison safety. After the trial court reinstated treatment over objection, the Louisiana Supreme Court stayed the order. It held that forcing drugs merely to facilitate execution "does not constitute medical treatment but is antithetical to the basic principles of the healing arts" and that doing so would violate the inmate's right to privacy and amount to cruel and unusual punishment under the Louisiana state constitution. Therefore, the state may not medicate incompetent death row prisoners over their objections simply for the purpose of restoring the prisoner to competence for execution.

ATKINS V. VIRGINIA, 536 U.S. 304 (2002)

Link to case: http://caselaw.lp.findlaw.com/scripts/getcase.pl?navby=case&
court=us&vol=536&page=304

Question: Does the Constitution prohibit the execution of a person with mental retardation?

Answer: Yes.

Daryl Atkins was convicted of murder and sentenced to death for abducting, robbing, and shooting a man. At the sentencing phase, the defense introduced a psychologist who testified that Atkins was mildly mentally retarded and had an IQ of 59. The Virginia Supreme Court affirmed the death sentence based on *Penry v. Lynaugh*, a 1989 U.S. Supreme Court case that allowed for the execution of individuals with mental retardation. In the *Atkins* case, the U.S. Supreme Court overruled this prior holding, now finding that executing mentally retarded prisoners was inconsistent with the "evolving standards of decency" that define what is considered "cruel and unusual punishment" under the Eighth Amendment. The Court noted that after the *Penry* case, a large number of states since 1989 had passed laws prohibiting the execution of the mentally retarded, and polls indicated that the majority of Americans were opposed to their execution. In addition, the Court reasoned that "executing the mentally retarded serves neither to deter others nor to mete out retribution appropriate for the lower level of culpability."

ROPER V. SIMMONS, 543 U.S. 551 (2005)

Link to case: http://caselaw.lp.findlaw.com/scripts/getcase.pl?navby=case&court=us&vol=543&page=551

Question: Does the Constitution prohibit the execution of an individual who committed a capital crime when he was under the age of 18?

Answer: Yes.

Christopher Simmons was 17 years old when he and an accomplice abducted a woman and threw her off a bridge to her death.

Mr. Simmons had planned the crime in advance, stating that he wanted to "murder someone," and then bragged about it afterward. Mr. Simmons was tried as an adult and sentenced to death. The Missouri Supreme Court affirmed the conviction and sentence. However, Mr. Simmons used the "evolving standards of decency" reasoning, as applied in the intervening U.S. Supreme Court decision in *Atkins v. Virginia* and filed a second appeal against Donald Roper, the superintendent of Potosi Correctional Center, with the Missouri Supreme Court. The Missouri court agreed with Mr. Simmons despite U.S. Supreme Court precedent in *Stanford v. Kentucky* that the minimum age for capital punishment was 16. In a 5–4 decision, The U.S. Supreme Court agreed with the Missouri court (and Mr. Simmons), holding that the execution of an individual for a crime committed before the age of 18 was a violation of the Eighth and Fourteenth Amendments. Similar to *Atkins*, the Court based its opinion on the fact that the majority of states (and international law) did not permit the execution of juveniles. The Court noted that the scientific community viewed adolescence as a period of poor decision making, developmental immaturity, and susceptibility to peer pressure, all of which rendered adolescents less culpable than adults and therefore not deserving of the ultimate penalty (i.e., death).

PANETTI V. QUARTERMAN, 551 U.S. 930 (2007)

Link to case: http://scholar.google.com/scholar_case?
case=2278250008123789539

Question: Are a "rational understanding" and a "factual awareness" necessary for a person to be found competent to be executed?

Answer: Yes.

Scott Panetti was sentenced to death for the murder of his estranged wife's parents. Mr. Panetti asked for a stay of execution, claiming that he was not competent to be executed. Nathaniel Quarterman was the director of the Correctional Institutions Division of the Texas Department of Criminal Justice. Mr. Panetti was examined, and the state court found him competent, without a hearing. On appeal, the U.S. Court of Appeals for the Fifth Circuit affirmed the finding, reasoning that although Mr. Panetti believed the real reason for his execution was to prevent him from preaching the gospel, he knew the state was executing him for murder. According to the court, this met the *Ford* standard for competency to be executed. The U.S. Supreme Court then reversed the Fifth Circuit holding. It stated that the *Ford* case required consideration of both Mr. Panetti's factual awareness that he was being executed and his "rational understanding" of the reasons for the execution. The Court also found that the procedures for evaluating Mr. Panetti's claim of incapacity were inadequate. However, the Court did not outline a specific standard for competency to be executed.

RYAN V. GONZALES, 568 U.S. 57 (2013)

Link: https://supreme.justia.com/cases/federal/us/568/57

Question: Does a death row inmate have the right to suspend federal habeas corpus proceedings when found incompetent to assist counsel?

Answer: No.

Ernest Valencia Gonzales was convicted of felony murder and sentenced to death for his repeated stabbing of Darrel and Deborah Wagner in front of their 7-year-old son during a burglary of the Wagners' home. Sean Carter was convicted by an Ohio jury of aggravated murder, aggravated robbery, and rape, and sentenced to death for anally raping his adoptive grandmother and stabbing her to death. In both cases the defendants filed habeas corpus proceedings. They were both found incompetent to stand trial at the time of these postconviction proceedings, and both requested and were granted a stay pending resolution of the competency question (Carter by the district court and Ryan by the Ninth Circuit Court of Appeal, overturning the lower court ruling). The Supreme Court granted certiorari in *Ryan v. Gonzales* to answer the same question posed in both cases. In a unanimous opinion, the Court reasoned that neither a statutory nor a constitutional right to competence exists during federal habeas corpus proceedings. Although the district court has broad discretion to grant a stay on habeas proceedings, in both cases, a stay was unwarranted because communication between the defendant and his attorney was unnecessary. The incompetence of the client had no significant impact on the attorney's ability to handle the habeas proceeding and the court record offered adequate enough information for counsel to proceed alone. Even if a decision by the district court found the competency of the client to be necessary, a stay of proceedings would only be warranted if the court found that the defendant was likely to regain competence in the foreseeable future. Without such a finding, a stay on federal habeas corpus proceedings would unreasonably burden the judicial system.

HALL V. FLORIDA, 134 S. CT. 1986 (2014)

Link to case: https://supreme.justia.com/cases/federal/us/572/12-10882/

Question: Is it a violation of the Constitution to rely upon a strict IQ score in determining intellectual disability for the purposes of death penalty proceedings?

Answer: Yes.

Freddie Lee Hall was sentenced to death for the murder of a pregnant woman. After the U.S. Supreme Court decided *Atkins*, Hall moved to vacate his sentence on the grounds that his intellectual disability exempted him from the death penalty. Hall failed to establish an IQ of 70 or below at his Atkins hearing, and thus, consistent with Florida's statutory requirement, he was incapable of satisfying Florida's intellectual disability standard. To prove intellectual disability under Florida law, a defendant must show

"significantly sub average general intellectual functioning"; it is statutorily defined as performance that is two or more standard deviations from
the mean score on a standardized intelligence test. Hall alleged that the
70-point IQ cutoff, articulated in the Florida's criminal code, violated the
Eighth and Fourteenth Amendments by creating an unacceptable risk that
persons with an intellectual disability will be executed.

The U.S. Supreme Court agreed. After reiterating its stance on the execution of the intellectually disabled, the Court then proceeded to determine how intellectual disability must be defined in order to implement
these principles and the holding of *Atkins*. The Court found that consensus among professionals was that an IQ score should be read not as a
single fixed number, but as a range. Therefore, Florida's mandatory cutoff
contravened professional practice in two ways: first, it left courts unable
to consider the additional evidence of medical and behavioral histories for
a defendant with an IQ above the cutoff; and second, the standard error
of measurement in each IQ test would remain unaccounted for due to
the mandatory cutoff. The Court also noted that only 9 states, at most,
mandated a strict IQ score cutoff at 70, and in 41 states, an individual in
Hall's position would not be deemed automatically eligible for the death
penalty. This, and other factors cited by the Court, offered strong evidence
of consensus that our society does not regard a 70-point cutoff as proper or
humane. Ultimately, the Court found it inappropriate to make one factor
"dispositive of a conjunctive and interrelated assessment" and therefore
held that "when a defendant's IQ test score falls within the test's acknowledged and inherent margin of error, the defendant must be able to present
additional evidence of intellectual disability, including testimony regarding
adaptive deficits."

MOORE V. TEXAS, 137 S. CT. 1039 (2017)

Link: https://www.supremecourt.gov/opinions/16pdf/15-797_n7io.pdf

Question: Does the Eighth Amendment proscribe the use of outdated medical standards for determining intellectual disability in death penalty cases?

Answer: Yes.

Bobby James Moore tried to rob a grocery store in Texas with two friends.
When a store employee screamed, Moore panicked and shot and instantly
killed a 71-year-old store clerk. Moore was sentenced to death. Moore,
who had an IQ of 74, appealed. The Texas Court of Appeals upheld Moore's
death sentence and said that in capital cases the state did not rely on a
medical definition of intellectual disability, but rather its own standards

in which the "consensus of Texas citizens" would decide who "should be exempted from the death penalty." The Supreme Court reversed the Texas appeals court and found that its use of an outdated medical definition of intellectual disability as well as outdated clinical guidelines for assessing adaptive functioning constituted a violation of the Eighth Amendment's prohibition against cruel and unusual punishment, as further explicated in prior Supreme Court cases (*Atkins* and *Hall*). In the Court opinion, Justice Ginsberg referenced Moore's developmental history, stating that at the age of 13, Moore lacked basic understanding of the days of the week, the months of the year, and the seasons. He could scarcely tell time or comprehend the standards of measure or the basic principle that subtraction is the reverse of addition. The Supreme Court did not specifically resolve which IQ tests should be considered, but described Moore as having an IQ score of 74, which, if adjusted for the standard error of measurement, yielded a range of 69 to 79. As established in *Hall v. Florida*, 134 S. Ct. 1986 (2014), since part of that range was under 70, the Texas court was required to move forward and consider Moore's adaptive functioning. The Supreme Court made clear that although the states have some flexibility in implementing *Atkins*, they do not have unfettered discretion, and that the medical community's current standards supply at least one constraint on a state's leeway.

MCWILLIAMS V. DUNN, 137 S. CT. 1790 (2017)

Link to case: https://www.leagle.com/decision/insco20170619e01

Question: Does *Ake v. Oklahoma* guarantee an indigent defendant access to expert psychiatric consultation not just at trial, but also if relevant to sentencing?

Answer: Yes.

James McWilliams, who sustained head injuries as a child and young adult, was an indigent defendant, sentenced to death by an Alabama judge, after being denied access to an independent expert who could have helped the defense understand and present his mental health issues. In *Ake v. Oklahoma*, the U.S. Supreme Court clearly recognized that once an indigent defendant has established that his mental health is likely to be a significant factor at trial, he is entitled to receive the assistance of an expert to assist his defense. The Court in *Ake* recognized that "such assistance is essential to providing the defendant 'a fair opportunity to present his defense,' and to ensuring that facts are resolved based on the views and expertise of 'psychiatrists for each party,' which is consistent with the adversary system."

In *McWilliams*, defense attorneys received a complex psychological report from the state's neuropsychologist 2 days before McWilliams sentencing hearing. The report stated that Mr. McWilliams had organic brain damage, genuine neuropsychological problems, and an obvious neuropsychological deficit, among other issues. The following day, Mr. McWilliams's defense team received his voluminous recent mental health records, and received his prison records on the day of the sentencing. The records showed, among other things, that Mr. McWilliams was being treated with psychotropic medication. A request for a continuance was denied, and McWilliams was inevitably sentenced to death.

The absence of an independent expert left Mr. McWilliams unable to present any mitigating evidence on his mental health—the only significant factor at his sentencing. The U.S. Supreme Court held that the state failed to meet its obligations under *Ake v. Oklahoma* to provide the defendant with access to a mental health expert to assist in evaluation, preparation, and presentation of a defense, including mitigation at sentencing. The Court mandated that once certain threshold matters, such as indigence and mental condition, are met, *Ake v. Oklahoma* clearly required that a defendant be provided with access to a competent mental health expert. The Court declined to address the question of whether *Ake* required that the state provide an indigent defendant with an expert retained specifically for the defense, as this case could be resolved on narrower grounds.

CHAPTER 27

ᴏᐯᴏ

Sex Offenders

LI-WEN G. LEE, HEATHER ELLIS CUCOLO,
AND JEREMY COLLEY

SPECHT V. PATTERSON, 386 U.S. 605 (1967)

Link to case: http://scholar.google.com/scholar_case?
case=3723552257968594646

Question: Can a person convicted under one statute be sentenced under a different statute without a new hearing?

Answer: No.

Francis Specht was convicted in Colorado for indecent liberties, a sex offense with a maximum 10-year sentence. Without notice and full hearing, he was sentenced under the Sex Offenders Act to an indeterminate term of 1 day to life. The act could be applied to convicted sex offenders found to be either a threat to the public if at large or a habitual offender and mentally ill. The procedure under the act required a psychiatric examination and report to be submitted to a court but did not include a full hearing. There was no opportunity to confront witnesses or to access hearsay evidence. Mr. Specht filed a habeas corpus petition for his release. Both the Colorado Supreme Court and then the U.S. Court of Appeals for the 10th Circuit rejected his petition. Mr. Specht then appealed to the U.S. Supreme Court. The Court held that commitment proceedings, whether civil or criminal, are still subject to the constitutional guarantees of the Fourteenth Amendment. The Court noted that the determination and sentencing under the act is a criminal punishment, despite its intention to prevent future harm rather than for retribution. As a result, due process

protections are required, including the presence of counsel and the opportunity to be heard, to be confronted with adverse witnesses, to cross-examine, and to offer evidence.

ALLEN V. ILLINOIS, 478 U.S. 364 (1986)

Link to case: http://scholar.google.com/scholar_case?
case=946918575027007848

Question: Does the Fifth Amendment protection against self-incrimination
apply to Illinois's Sexual Dangerous Persons Act?

Answer: No.

Terry Allen was charged in Illinois with unlawful restraint and deviant
sexual assault. The state sought to have him found a sexually dangerous
person under the Illinois Sexually Dangerous Persons Act, a finding that
requires proving the existence of a mental disorder for more than 1 year
and a propensity to commit sexual assaults. In accordance with the Act,
two psychiatrists examined Mr. Allen and testified at trial. He was found
to be a sexually dangerous person and then appealed on the basis that
the psychiatric testimony included information elicited from him in violation of his privilege against self-incrimination. The Appellate Court
of Illinois for the Third District agreed with Mr. Allen, but the Supreme
Court of Illinois upheld the determination. The U.S. Supreme Court then
heard the case and agreed with the state. It found that although the Act
could be applied only if criminal charges were already filed, the Act itself
was not criminal—but civil—in nature, because the goal was to provide
treatment rather than punishment. It found that the provision of care in a
maximum security facility also providing care to convicts did not establish
punishment over treatment. In addition, the provision of some due process safeguards by the act did not turn the act into a criminal proceeding
requiring the full range of due process protections. The Court further
noted that the Fourteenth Amendment guarantee of due process does not
require application of the Fifth Amendment privilege against self-incrimination in civil proceedings.

MATTER OF PERSONAL RESTRAINT OF YOUNG, 857 P.2D 989 (WASH.1993)

Link to case: https://law.justia.com/cases/washington/supreme-court/
1993/57837-1-1.html

Question: Is the Washington State sexually violent predator statute a criminal law?

Answer: No.

Andre Brigham Young was incarcerated after conviction for rape, and he had a history of committing other rapes. One day prior to his release, the state filed for commitment under the Washington sexually violent predator statute, the Community Protection Act of 1990. Vance Russell Cunningham was convicted of an unrelated rape; he also had a history of committing prior sexual offenses. In Mr. Cunningham's case, the state filed for commitment several months after he had been released from prison. Mr. Young and Mr. Cunningham appealed to the Supreme Court of Washington and argued that the statute violated the double jeopardy clause and the prohibition against ex post facto laws. The court concluded that the statute was civil and that therefore the criminal protections of double jeopardy and ex post facto laws did not apply. It noted that commitment requires a mental disorder leading to the commission of violent sexual offenses and that committed persons are treated in a psychiatric facility and released as soon as they are no longer dangerous. Mr. Young and Mr. Cunningham also argued that substantive and procedural due process were violated in a number of ways. On these issues, the court found that a defendant must be permitted to appear in court within 72 hours to contest probable cause, the state was required to show acute dangerousness for defendants not incarcerated, least restrictive alternatives must be considered, and jury unanimity was required at the beyond a reasonable doubt threshold.

KANSAS V. HENDRICKS, 521 U.S. 346 (1997)

Link to case: http://scholar.google.com/scholar_case?case=3660172212792959574

Question: Does the procedure for civil commitment established by the Kansas Sexually Violent Predator (SVP) Act violate principles of due process, double jeopardy, and ex post facto?

Answer: No.

Leroy Hendricks was convicted of taking indecent liberties with two 13-year-old boys and was then incarcerated. Shortly before his release, the state sought to confine civilly Mr. Hendricks as a sexually violent predator under the Kansas SVP Act. During his trial to determine whether he qualified as a sexually violent predator, Mr. Hendricks testified about his lengthy history of sexual offenses against children. He further admitted to abusing children whenever not confined, and while he expressed the hope to not offend against children again, he stated that the only guarantee was "to die." He agreed with the diagnosis of pedophilia, acknowledged that he was not cured, and further opined that the treatment was ineffective. He was found to be a sexually violent predator and to have a "mental abnormality" qualifying him for confinement under the act. Mr. Hendricks claimed that the act violated the due process, double jeopardy, and ex post facto clauses of the Constitution. The Kansas Supreme Court agreed that "mental abnormality" did not meet the standard of a mental illness for involuntary commitment purposes; the State of Kansas appealed to the U.S. Supreme Court. The Court reversed the appellate decision by ruling that the definition of "mental abnormality" in the Act satisfied "substantive" due process requirements in that there is no constitutional basis for any particular definition of mental disorder nor specific nomenclature. The specific term "mental illness" is not required. The Court further found that lack of effective treatment did not make the Act functionally criminal (as opposed to civil) and therefore an unconstitutional violation of the prohibition against double jeopardy and ex post facto principles.

MCKUNE V. LILE, 536 U.S. 24 (2002)

Link to case: http://scholar.google.com/scholar_case?
case=16143402596203476658

Question: Does incentivizing participation during incarceration in the Kansas Sexual Abuse Treatment Program (SATP), which requires admitting past offenses, violate the Fifth Amendment privilege against self-incrimination?

Answer: No.

Robert Lile was convicted of rape, aggravated sodomy, and aggravated kidnapping despite his claim that the sexual activity was consensual. Before release from prison, he was ordered to participate in the SATP, which requires discussion and acceptance of responsibility of the crime(s) of conviction as well as details of prior sexual activities, including uncharged criminal offenses. This information is not privileged, although at the time Mr. Lile's case was heard, there was no incriminating evidence released under the SATP. Refusal to participate in the program would result in loss of certain privileges and transfer to a maximum security prison. Mr. Lile refused to participate on the grounds that the consequences of nondisclosure were so significant that they constituted compelled self-incrimination that would violate his Fifth Amendment privilege. He sought an injunction to prevent loss of privileges and transfer to a more secure facility. The district court agreed about the Fifth Amendment violation claim, and the U.S. Court of Appeals for the Tenth Circuit affirmed. The U.S. Supreme Court did not agree, however, and found that the program did not violate Mr. Lile's Fifth Amendment right as along as (1) the program served a legitimate penological objective, (2) the consequences also had a rehabilitative function (i.e., teach that actions have consequences), and (3) the consequences were not so severe as to be coercive.

KANSAS V. CRANE, 534 U.S. 407 (2002)

Link to case: http://scholar.google.com/scholar_case?case=11856713111605024563

Question: Does the ruling in *Kansas v. Hendricks* require the state to prove that a dangerous individual is completely unable to control his behavior?

Answer: No.

Michael Crane was convicted of a sexual offense, and the state pursued civil commitment hearings under the Kansas SVP Act. A psychiatric witness for the state diagnosed him with exhibitionism and antisocial personality disorder, and the trial court ordered his commitment without a finding regarding whether he could control his dangerous behavior. Mr. Crane's commitment was overturned on appeal to the Kansas Supreme Court based on a ruling that Mr. Crane did not meet the *Hendricks* requirement of proof that a dangerous individual is completely unable to control his behavior. Kansas appealed to the U.S. Supreme Court with the argument that the interpretation of the appellate court was too rigid. The U.S. Supreme Court determined that a complete lack of control was not necessary to be committed as a sexually violent predator. However, the Court disagreed with Kansas and found that some volitional criteria was required in order to distinguish dangerous offenders subject to civil commitment from those appropriately addressed exclusively through criminal proceedings. Because lack of control is not demonstrable with "mathematical precision," the Court noted that serious difficulty controlling behavior was adequate for SVP determinations.

SMITH V. DOE, 538 U.S. 84 (2003)

Link to case: https://supreme.justia.com/cases/federal/us/538/84/

Question: Does Alaska's Sex Offender Registration Act violate the Ex Post Facto Clause?

Answer: No.

In 1994, the Alaska Sex Offender Registration Act ("Act") was passed by state legislators concerned with the rise of sex crimes. The Act requires all convicted sex offenders to register with the state. The Act also mandates that the offender's name, aliases, address, photograph, physical description, driver's license number, motor vehicle identification numbers, place of employment, date of birth, crime, date and place of conviction, length and conditions of sentence, and a statement as to whether the offender is in compliance, be published on the Internet and available for public viewing for all purposes. Both the Act's registration and notification requirements are retroactive.

Respondents, John Doe I and John Doe II were convicted of aggravated sex offenses. Both men were released from prison about five years before the act passed. The respondents, along with the wife of one of them, brought an action under 42 U.S. C. §1983, seeking to declare the Act void as to them under, inter alia, the Ex Post Facto Clause, U.S. Const., Art. I, §10, cl. 1.

The Ninth Circuit found that the effects of the Act were punitive but the U.S. Supreme Court disagreed. In a 6-3 decision, the Supreme Court held that the sex offender registry was not punishment and therefore the Alaska Sex Offender Registration Act was nonpunitive. The majority determined that Alaska had implemented a "civil regulatory scheme," not a criminal procedure. Because the regulatory scheme is simply a series of civil laws designed to protect the public, its retroactive application does not violate the Ex Post Facto Clause.

That same year (2003) the US Supreme Court held that the Connecticut sex offender registry statute, which predicated registration on conviction alone, and not further findings of dangerousness, was not an unconstitutional deprivation of due process. The Court declined to decide whether or not the statute implicated other constitutional issues (e.g., liberty interests in avoiding public disclosure). (*Connecticut Department of Public Safety v. Doe*).

U.S. V. COMSTOCK, 560 U.S. 126 (2010)

Link to case: https://supreme.justia.com/cases/federal/us/560/126/

Question: Can Congress enact legislation to commit civilly convicted, mentally ill, sexually violent federal prisoners beyond their schedule release date?

Answer: Yes.

In 2006, the U.S. government instituted postincarceration civil commitment proceedings against five men convicted of sexual offenses. Three of the men had been charged with possession of child pornography, and the other two with sexual abuse of a minor. The government sought to confine them pursuant to Federal Statute 4248, which allowed for the indefinite confinement of mentally ill, sexually dangerous federal prisoners beyond the date they would otherwise be released, with "mental illness" defined as having a disorder that would make it difficult to refrain from "sexually violent conduct or child molestation." The men opposed their commitment, making double jeopardy, ex post facto, equal protection, and due process claims (including that the standard of proof should be beyond a reasonable doubt). They also claimed that Congress had exceeded its powers in enacting the civil commitment statute. The district court dismissed the case, and the U.S. Court of Appeals for the Fourth Circuit affirmed the dismissal. The U.S. Supreme Court granted certiorari about the congressional power issue and found that Congress had the power to enact this civil commitment statute. It noted that while the scope of the federal government was restricted by the Constitution, Congress did have the power to enact legislation that was "necessary and proper" and "rationally related" to the implementation of a constitutionally enumerated power (see Article I of the Constitution), in this case continuing a long-standing policy of providing care and control of individuals who may be at risk to third parties.

DOES #1–5 V. SNYDER, 834 F.3D 696 (2016)

Link to case: https://www.leagle.com/decision/infco20160825100

Question: Must there be evidence as to the effectiveness of a sex offender registry to reduce recidivism and protect public safety for it to be constitutional?

Answer: Yes.

Michigan passed the Sex Offender Registration Act (SORA) in 1994, initially as a nonpublic list of registered sex offenders used strictly by law enforcement. Over the next two decades, the reach of SORA expanded dramatically, so that the registry not only became public but prohibited those on the list from living, working, or loitering within 1,000 feet of schools. The plaintiffs in this case, who filed anonymously, argued that various provisions of SORA were unconstitutionally vague, should not be enforced under strict liability standards, infringed upon freedom of speech, and

hobbled their rights to parent, work, and travel. The Sixth Circuit found
the retroactive application of the Michigan SORA to be punitive and therefore unconstitutional. In conducting the rationality-excessiveness test, the
court considered the legislature's stated goals of promoting public safety
and reducing recidivism. The court found little to no evidence on the record
to support the claim that SORA served either of these goals. Considering
the stated goal of reducing recidivism, the court found the evidence on the
record demonstrated SORA had, at best, no impact on recidivism. In fact,
the court found evidence in the record that the law may actually *increase*
the risk of recidivism.

Compounding the court's unwillingness to uphold SORA was the State
of Michigan's failure to so much as analyze recidivism rates in the state,
despite having the necessary data to do so. As for public safety, the court
found that the record disclosed no relationship between SORA's registration requirements and public safety whatsoever. To uphold SORA, the
court found, would amount to writing a blank check to the legislature to
pass whatever laws it wished.

Of note was the unique approach that the Sixth Circuit took by discussing
"scientific evidence that refutes moralized judgments about sex offenders,
specifically that they pose a unique and substantial risk of recidivism," fo-
cusing on the implication of the court's suspicion of the long-held belief
that sex offender recidivism was "frightening and high" and that it was not
clearly supported by the scientific evidence.

MILLARD V. RANKIN, 265 F.SUPP.3D 1211 (2017)

Link to case: https://www.leagle.com/decision/infdco20170901c12

Question: Must the restrictions of a state sex offender registry be proportional to the original commitment offense so as not to violate the Eighth
Amendment?

Answer: Yes.

People registered under the Colorado Sex Offender Registration Act (SORA)
brought a § 1983 civil action and claimed that SORA violated their rights
under the Eighth and Fourteenth Amendments to the U.S. Constitution.
In finding that the plaintiffs' rights were violated, the court reviewed the
personal hardships faced by the plaintiffs, in particular, the ostracization
by the community, and prevention of assimilation back into society. The
court emphasized the continued punishment by the community through a
connection between the case at bar and a recent U.S. Supreme Court ruling

on privacy and access to the Internet by registered offenders: *Packingham v. North Carolina*, 137 S. Ct. 1730, 1731, 198 L. Ed. 2d 273 (U.S. 2017).

In *Packingham*, the U.S. Supreme Court held that a North Carolina statute that made it a felony for a registered sex offender to knowingly access a commercial social networking website that permits minor children to become members or to create or maintain personal web pages, impermissibly restricted lawful speech in violation of the First Amendment. Although *Packingham* had dealt with First Amendment violations of registered sex offenders, it contained a foreshadowing statement that applied directly to the issue in *Millard*. In his majority opinion in *Packingham*, Justice Kennedy highlighted the troubling fact that the law imposes severe restrictions on persons who already have served their sentence and are no longer subject to the supervision of the criminal justice system, but noted that this was not an issue currently before the Court.

Two months after the decision in *Packingham*, the *Millard* court seized upon the significance of Justice Kennedy's observation and took advantage of the ripeness of that issue in the case at bar. The *Millard* court fittingly took the language contained in *Packingham* and applied it to the relevant facts and circumstances of the *Millard* plaintiffs to conclude that they suffered continued punishment in the community that was disproportionate to the offenses they committed. According to the Court, SORA mimicked historical forms of punishment and thus its effects were punitive and violated the Eighth Amendment and the plaintiffs' substantive and procedural due process rights.

CHAPTER 28

Questions on Criminal Law
and Incarceration

QUESTIONS

1. In its decision in *North Carolina v. Alford*, the U.S. Supreme Court affirmed which of the following statements?
   A. The Fourteenth Amendment requires that defendants retain their right to a guilty plea despite the advice of competent counsel.
   B. Mens rea need not be considered in cases of clearly premeditated murder.
   C. If the principal motivation behind a guilty plea is fear of death, the plea is invalidated.
   D. The standard for a plea is whether that plea is a "voluntary and intelligent" choice among one's options.
   E. Because the local North Carolina court issued the incorrect jury instructions, Alford's guilty plea should not have been accepted.

2. The U.S. Supreme Court has ruled that executing juveniles or the mentally retarded is a violation of which constitutional amendment?
   A. First
   B. Fifth
   C. Sixth
   D. Eighth
   E. Fourteenth

3. Which of the following statements is most accurate regarding diminished capacity defenses?
   A. They are required by the Due Process Clause of the U.S. Constitution.
   B. They cannot be advanced by pro se defendants.

C. They are unrelated to issues of intent and mens rea.

D. Their use and relevance are the purview of each state.

E. They are unavailable to defendants opting for trial by jury.

4. A frequently cited basis for U.S. Supreme Court decisions finding that involuntary, postincarceration sexually violent predator commitment programs do not constitute criminal sanctions is:

A. Involuntary commitments do not extend past the period of parole supervision after incarceration mandated during the sentencing phase of the criminal proceedings.

B. Involuntary commitment is for the purpose of treatment rather than punishment.

C. Involuntary commitment is for those individuals convicted of sexual offenses who failed to complete sex offender treatment during incarceration.

D. Convicted sex offenders have both committed criminal acts and suffer from a mental disorder and therefore require both punishment and treatment.

E. Involuntary commitment requires a showing that sexual offense recidivism is more likely than not after release from incarceration.

5. Does the U.S. Constitution require that a mentally ill prisoner receive a judicial hearing before he receives treatment over objection?

A. Yes. Mentally ill convicted prisoners need to be protected from prison-associated health care professionals, and a judicial hearing is therefore necessary to adjudicate treatment over objection.

B. No. Mentally ill convicted prisoners do not have the right to refuse medically appropriate treatment.

C. No. Mentally ill convicted prisoners have the right to refuse treatment, but an administrative review by medical professionals of the treatment refusal and the need for treatment over objection is sufficient to satisfy due process.

D. Yes. Prisoners with mental illness are entitled to the same due process rights as individuals who are involuntarily committed to civilian hospitals.

6. The U.S. Supreme Court has ruled that a state is able to makes laws that:

A. Punish people addicted to drugs with incarceration

B. Punish people addicted to drugs with incarceration followed by forced treatment

C. Force people addicted to drugs to undergo treatment

D. Increase incarceration times for people addicted to drugs if they break another law

E. Treat people addicted to drugs exactly as people who are not

7. Which of the following best illustrates the U.S. Supreme Court's use of the concept of an "evolving standard of decency"?
   A. *Roper v. Simmons* ruling against precedent set in *Stanford v. Kentucky*
   B. *Payne v. Tennessee* ruling against precedent set in *Booth v. Maryland*
   C. *Ford v. Wainwright* decision in keeping with the history of common law
   D. None of the above

8. *U.S. v. Comstock*, a case involving the civil commitment of a sex offender, was decided on the basis of:
   A. Procedural due process
   B. Substantive due process
   C. Double jeopardy
   D. Equal protection
   E. Congressional authority

9. What is the legal burden of proof in competence to stand trial hearings in federal court?
   A. Clear and convincing evidence
   B. Beyond a reasonable doubt
   C. Without due cause
   D. Preponderance of the evidence

10. In cases of extreme emotional disturbance (EED), the burden of proving the EED:
    A. Is typically only to a preponderance of the evidence because these cases are normally civil in nature
    B. Is a presumption in a criminal case and so needs to be proved in the negative by the state to beyond a reasonable doubt
    C. Is closely related to whether the defendant is proposing a not guilty by reason of insanity plea
    D. Can constitutionally rest upon the defendant
    E. Need only apply if the murder occurred in the setting of a different violent crime, such as robbery

11. In Miranda v. Arizona, the primary reason given by the Court in establishing the affirmative need for the police to inform suspects of their rights was:
    A. Many defendants have borderline intelligence.
    B. First-time defendants cannot be assumed to know their rights.
    C. The application of specific constitutional rights varies from case to case.
    D. The inherently coercive nature of being in police custody
    E. Defendants are presumed incompetent to stand trial until proved otherwise.

12. A psychiatrist is asked by the prosecution to evaluate a capital defendant for competency to stand trial and to form an opinion about the defendant's future risk for dangerousness in case of a capital sentencing hearing. There is no notice given to defense counsel, and the psychiatrist does not explain the limits of confidentiality. According to the ruling in *Estelle v. Smith*, which best describes the way in which this defendant's constitutional rights have been violated?
    A. Fifth Amendment, because he did not know he could refuse, *and* Eighth Amendment, because prosecution is seeking the death penalty in a defendant who may not be competent for trial
    B. Sixth Amendment, because he did not know he could refuse examination
    C. Fifth Amendment, because he did not have access to counsel, *and* Sixth Amendment, because he did not know he could refuse
    D. Fifth Amendment, because he did not know he could refuse, *and* Sixth Amendment, because he did not have access to counsel
    E. Fifth Amendment, because he did not have access to counsel

13. Prior to the Insanity Defense Reform Act of 1984, if there was some evidence of mental illness, the burden of proof in federal court was on:
    A. The government to prove sanity beyond a reasonable doubt
    B. The government to prove sanity by preponderance of the evidence
    C. The defendant to prove insanity beyond a reasonable doubt
    D. The defendant to prove insanity by clear and convincing evidence.

14. Consideration of competency at any time during a trial when sufficient doubt arises as to a defendant's current competence protects the defendant's right to:
    A. A fair trial
    B. Autonomy
    C. Freedom of speech
    D. Immunity

15. During participation in a sexual offender treatment program, the Fifth Amendment privilege against self-incrimination is:
    A. Protected by allowing persons to participate even if they have not acknowledged their offense(s) or provided a sexual history
    B. Protected by guaranteeing that disclosed information cannot be shared outside of treatment
    C. Not guaranteed because there is a legitimate goal of rehabilitation
    D. Not relevant because treatment occurs outside of the criminal justice system

16. Which of the following statements is most accurate regarding the Supreme Court's holding in *Montana v Egelhoff*?
    A. Voluntary intoxication was deemed a necessary consideration in criminal cases.
    B. The holding is not important to most jurisdictions, so it has had minimal impact on subsequent case law and practice.
    C. All states must offer charged defendants the option of pleading not guilty by reason of insanity.
    D. It affirmed that jurisdictions can constitutionally preclude consideration of voluntary intoxication when trying a criminal defendant.
    E. All evidence, regardless of probative value, is required to be entertained by the trier of fact.

17. Which of the following statements is true?
    A. American Academy of Psychiatry and the Law (AAPL) ethical guidelines prohibit a psychiatrist from providing psychiatric treatment to a patient found incompetent to be executed.
    B. AAPL ethical guidelines prohibit psychiatrists from conducting examinations of competency to be sentenced in capital cases.
    C. American Medical Association (AMA) guidelines state that physicians should not participate in executions.
    D. American Psychiatric Association (APA) guidelines prohibit a psychiatrist from providing psychiatric treatment to a patient found incompetent to be executed.
    E. The AMA states that testifying to medical aspects of aggravating or mitigating circumstances during the sentencing phase of a capital case constitutes physician participation in an execution.

18. The standard for a confession to be admissible is:
    A. Voluntary and knowing
    B. Informed consent
    C. Clear and convincing
    D. Competent
    E. Intelligent

19. What U.S. Supreme Court case first defined the criteria for competency to stand trial?
    A. *Drope v. Missouri*
    B. *Jackson v. Indiana*
    C. *Dusky v. U.S.*
    D. *Wilson v. U.S.*

20. An indigent defendant seeks to put forth an insanity defense, but the state denies his request to provide a psychiatric expert to examine his mental state at the time of the crime. According to *Ake v. Oklahoma*, what constitutional right has been violated?
    A. Fifth Amendment
    B. Sixth Amendment
    C. Eighth Amendment
    D. Fourteenth Amendment Due Process Clause
    E. Fourteenth Amendment Equal Protection Clause

21. Which of the following statements is most accurate regarding the decision of the Washington, D.C. Court of Appeals in *Ibn-Tamas v. U.S.*?
    A. The "battered wife syndrome" is clearly a legitimate clinical entity and so should be considered by courts in cases involving alleged abuse.
    B. The "battered wife syndrome" is clearly not a legitimate clinical entity and so should not be considered by courts in cases involving alleged abuse.
    C. Expert testimony regarding the "battered wife syndrome" may be admissible, depending on the credentials of the expert and whether the testimony's probative value exceeds its potential prejudicial impact.
    D. The defense erred in selecting a psychologist as the expert because "battered wife syndrome" is more accurately placed in the purview of psychiatrists.
    E. Clearly established victims of "battered wife syndrome" should have immediate and full exculpation if their violence was against the historical abuser.

22. Which of the following reasons has led courts to find sex offender registration laws in violation of the Eighth Amendment?
    A. The offenders already spent time in prison.
    B. The restrictions imposed on registered sex offenders were disproportionate to their crimes.
    C. There was no evidence presented that registration process accomplished another goal, such as reducing recidivism.
    D. The registration rationale was based on irrational fear.
    E. All of the above

23. The three-judge panel convened for *Brown v. Plata* to remedy the violation of prisoners' rights related to proper medical and mental health care was authorized under which congressional act?
    A. Employee Retirement Income Security Act (ERISA)
    B. Health Insurance Portability and Accountability Act (HIPPA)

C. Prison Litigation Reform Act (PLRA)
D. Mental Health Parity Act
E. The Act of 1812

24. A successful diminished capacity defense:
    A. Can transfer a case from criminal to civil domain
    B. Frequently leads to full acquittal of charge
    C. Can be affirmatively placed despite clear lack of competence
    D. Can reduce a specific intent crime to a general intent crime
    E. Can originate from the prosecution

25. Mental disorder considerations in SVP commitment proceedings:
    A. Must be linked to sexually offending behaviors
    B. Are defined by the term "mental illness"
    C. Do not include personality disorders
    D. Are required to satisfy "procedural" due process requirements

26. A prison official who knowingly places a prisoner in a situation where the official is aware of a substantial risk of serious harm may be held liable for acting with:
    A. Nonmaleficence
    B. Deliberate indifference
    C. Failure to provide a comfortable environment
    D. Negligence
    E. Indifference

27. Which of the following cases addressed the issue of a mentally ill person's competence to be executed?
    A. *Atkins v. Virginia*
    B. *Roper v. Simmons*
    C. *Estelle v. Smith*
    D. *State v. Perry*
    E. *Ford v. Wainwright*

28. Which of the following statements is true regarding the involuntary treatment of a death row inmate with antipsychotic medication to restore his competence to be executed?
    A. The APA prohibits treatment of capital defendants who are incompetent to stand trial.
    B. In *State v. Perry*, the U.S. Supreme Court found that involuntary treatment with medication to restore competency represented cruel and unusual punishment.
    C. Federal law dictates that when an offender is convicted of a capital crime, he no longer maintains privacy rights that would allow him to refuse medical treatment.

D. *Washington v. Harper* specifically addressed antipsychotic treatment refusal in death row inmates and found that it is unconstitutional for the state to treat over objection for the purpose of restoring competency.

E. In *State v. Perry*, the court reasoned that forcing drugs merely to facilitate execution does not constitute medical treatment and instead violates the inmate's right to privacy and constitutes cruel and unusual punishment.

29. The holding in *Colorado v. Connelly* found no mental health exception to the existing standard that a confession taken from police interrogation should only be suppressed if:

A. *Miranda* rights were not presented prior to the confession.

B. There was coercive police activity used in obtaining the police confession.

C. The confession was not the product of "a rational intellect and free will."

D. There was illegal search and seizure prior to the police interrogation.

E. It is not promptly notarized following the confession.

31. In *Vitek v. Jones*, the transfer of Mr. Jones to a mental hospital was declared unconstitutional because:

A. It infringed on his rights prohibiting cruel and unusual punishment.

B. It infringed on his right to due process under the Fourteenth Amendment.

C. He was forced to acknowledge his mental illness.

D. The receiving facility was unable to care for his basic medical needs.

32. The constitutional challenge to the procedure of police confessions in *Colorado v. Connelly* rests on which U.S. constitutional amendment?

A. First

B. Second

C. Fourth

D. Eighth

E. Fourteenth

33. Which of the following was a consideration in the decision in *Atkins v. Virginia*?

A. Mental retardation does not affect an individual's culpability.

B. Execution of mentally retarded offenders would provide a reasonable deterrent effect for other potential offenders with mental retardation.

C. Mentally retarded offenders may be less able to assist in their defense.

D. Very few states prohibit the execution of mentally retarded offenders.

34. Proof of lack of ability to control behavior in SVP commitment is:
    A. Not required if mental disorder or equivalent is shown because of the implied influence of mental disorder on volitional behavior
    B. Not required if the criminal history indicates repeated serious recidivistic behavior
    C. Required because there is a clear demarcation between emotional and volitional behavior
    D. Adequately established if there is proof of serious difficulty controlling behavior

35. Which of the following is not necessarily a reason that amnesia may render a defendant incompetent?
    A. Inability to follow the proceedings
    B. Inability to discuss proceedings rationally with an attorney
    C. Inability to remember all details of the alleged crime
    D. Ability to testify on one's own behalf

36. What additional factor was added to the definition of the "deliberate indifference" standard in *Farmer v. Brennan*?
    A. Negligence
    B. Actual awareness of the risk of serious harm
    C. Disregard of the risk of harm
    D. Physical injury

37. Which of the following statements is true concerning the use of victim impact statements as decided in *Payne v. Tennessee*?
    A. Victim impact statements aid the jury in assessing moral culpability.
    B. Psychiatrists are prohibited from testifying about the psychological impact of a crime on the victim's family.
    C. The jury should decide a capital sentence based only on the character of the defendant and the circumstances of the crime.
    D. Victim impact statements contribute to arbitrary or capricious sentencing.
    E. The state does not have a legitimate interest in rebutting the mitigating evidence offered by the defense.

38. Which of the following NGRI defenses is most likely to succeed in a *M'Naghten* jurisdiction?
    A. A patient with obsessive-compulsive disorder who assaults someone on the street when an outdoor merchant attempts to sell her a piece of luggage she thinks is full of germs
    B. A patient with posttraumatic stress disorder who shoots his girlfriend believing he was in the battlefield facing an undercover enemy combatant

C. A patient with pathological gambling who could not stop himself from spending his employer's money at the casino

D. A patient with pedophilic disorder who repeatedly masturbates in a children's park

39. The "necessary and proper" clause under which the statute in *U.S. v. Comstock* was determined to be constitutional can be found in which amendment?
   A. First
   B. Fifth
   C. Eighth
   D. Fourteenth
   E. None of the above

40. Mr. Dean, who has a history of schizoaffective disorder, went into a restaurant and shot all of the meat-eating diners. He was acutely psychotic at the time of the crime. In an ALI jurisdiction, which would he have to argue in order to get an NGRI verdict?
   A. At the time of the crime he believed that eating meat was morally wrong.
   B. At the time of the crime he was hearing auditory hallucinations telling him that God believes eating meat is wrong, and God was telling him to kill meat eaters in order to save these people from contracting and spreading deadly meat-borne illnesses.
   C. At the time of the crime he believed that people who eat meat should be shot just like the animals that are shot for food.
   D. At the time of the crime he believed his law breaking in the service of social activism should be exculpatory.

41. The U.S. Supreme Court ruled that it is unconstitutional for a state to regulate drug abuse through:
   A. Criminal sanctions against the unauthorized manufacture, prescription, sale, purchase, or possession of narcotics within its borders
   B. Compulsory treatment for those addicted to narcotics, with periods of involuntary confinement as part of a treatment program
   C. Penal sanctions for a failure to comply with established compulsory treatment procedures
   D. Public health education and efforts to ameliorate the economic and social conditions under which drug abuse flourishes
   E. Imprisonment of an addict who travels through a state's jurisdiction

42. Legal challenges raised regarding commitment in SVP programs include:
    A. Double jeopardy
    B. Ex post facto lawmaking
    C. Substantive and procedural due process
    D. Fifth Amendment privilege against self-incrimination
    E. All of the above

43. In *People v. Patterson*, the New York Court of Appeals proposed which of the following arguments in its support of state law as it existed governing extreme emotional disturbance (EED) defenses?
    A. The law still required the state to prove all elements of the crime, despite placing the burden of proving the EED on the defense.
    B. The law had passed by a resounding majority in the senate and so should be offered wide latitude in interpretation.
    C. Because it was a state and not a federal law, it was not governed by the U.S. Constitution.
    D. Voluntary intoxication has always been accepted in common law and so should be incorporated into EED considerations.
    E. As a fundamental right, access to an EED defense is firmly rooted in the U.S. Constitution.

44. The case of *Powell v. Texas* (392 U.S. 514, 1968) led to the U.S. Supreme Court review of a statute for the alleged infliction of a cruel and unusual punishment. In this case, the Court ruled that Mr. Powell was rightfully convicted for:
    A. Being an alcoholic
    B. Being drunk in public
    C. Committing a murder while drunk
    D. Performing an unlawful act while drunk that was the product of a mental disease of defect
    E. Being unable to tell right from wrong when drunk

45. Can a pretrial detainee be treated over his objection for the purpose of restoring competence to stand trial?
    A. Yes, as long as the court finds that the patient is also dangerous.
    B. Yes, but only if certain criteria about medical appropriateness and governmental interests are met.
    C. No. Forcible medication can only be given against someone's will for purposes of treatment, not for competence to stand trial.
    D. No. Medications can never be given to a pretrial detainee against his will because the side effects might result in unfair trial prejudice.

46. Which of the following was cited as a reason to hold defendants to a different standard of competence for pro se representation than for competency to stand trial in *Indiana v. Edwards*?
    A. Mentally ill defendants are always incompetent.
    B. The variable quality of court-appointed legal personnel
    C. The need to affirm the dignity of the defendant
    D. The inherent inequality of the U.S. legal system

47. *Brown v. Plata* involves a class of prisoners in California who:
    A. Alleged sexual abuse
    B. Alleged wrongful conviction
    C. Had serious medical problems
    D. Had serious mental health problems
    E. Had serious medical and/or mental health problems

48. Sex offender treatment programs during incarceration:
    A. Should not predicate prison privileges on program participation
    B. May require participants to take responsibility for the sexual offense leading to conviction
    C. Do not consider past sexual behaviors not associated with formal criminal history to be relevant
    D. Must be made available to those individuals who may be subject to SVP commitments

49. In evaluating whether someone is ineligible for the death penalty due to an intellectual disability, a clinician should:
    A. Read the IQ score as a range instead of a single fixed number
    B. Consider the additional evidence of medical and behavioral histories for a defendant
    C. Provide testimony regarding adaptive deficits
    D. All of the above

50. In a capital murder case, an expert who testifies about characteristics that might increase the likelihood of future dangerousness should:
    A. Inform the jury that predictions of future dangerousness can be made precisely and with absolute certainty
    B. Include the defendant's race or ethnicity as a factor that contributes to increased risk
    C. Make sure to root his or her opinion in evidence-based practice standards, including data from standardized risk assessment tools
    D. Testify that the vast majority of people who are violent suffer from mental illnesses

ANSWERS

1. **D**

The U.S. Supreme Court, in its landmark decision in *North Carolina v. Alford*, held that Mr. Alford's plea, despite his protestation of innocence, was appropriate because he was well counseled and had ample evidence supporting his guilt. It constituted a "knowing and intelligent" choice between the alternatives. The Court therefore felt that his guilty plea (which has since come to be known as an "Alford plea") was appropriately accepted by the lower court. One's right to a guilty plea is independent from the advice of counsel. Mens rea is a critical consideration in cases of murder. The *Alford* case refuted the contention that fear of death should invalidate a guilty plea. There were no issues of faulty jury instructions in the case.

2. **D**

The Eighth Amendment protects against "cruel and unusual punishment." The U.S. Supreme Court cited the Eighth Amendment in holding that executing mentally retarded defendants (*Atkins v. Virginia*) or defendants who were juveniles at the time of their crime (*Roper v. Simmons*) is unconstitutional. The First Amendment protects freedom of speech. The Fifth Amendment provides the right to protection against self-incrimination. The Sixth Amendment provides the right to counsel. The Due Process Clause of the Fourteenth Amendment is used by the federal judiciary to make the Bill of Rights applicable to the states, and the Equal Protection Clause requires each state to provide equal protection under the law to similar classes of people in its jurisdiction.

3. **D**

Diminished capacity defenses can, among other things, reduce a specific intent conviction (murder) to a general intent conviction (manslaughter). Because it is an affirmative defense, it originates with the defendant, not the prosecutor. It is unrelated to jurisdiction of charge and requires a competent defendant. While it is possible that a diminished capacity defense can lead to full charge acquittal (e.g., if there were no lesser charges based on the diminished capacity), this is rarely the case.

4. **B**

The decisions in *Allen v. Illinois*, 478 U.S. 364 (1986), *In re Young and Cunningham*, 857 P.2d 989 (1993), and *Kansas v. Hendricks*, 521 U.S. 346 (1997) cite, in part, the goal of treatment. The role of treatment, even if in conjunction with incapacitation or as an ancillary goal, establishes sexually violent predator statutes as nonpunitive in nature and therefore subject to standards for civil, rather than criminal, proceedings. Commitments may extend until there is a showing that the confined person is no longer dangerous, independent of the duration of criminal sanctions. Completion, or not, of sex offender treatment during incarceration may be a consideration in mental abnormality and dangerousness considerations, but neither the SVP statutes nor court decisions specifically cite failure to complete sex offender treatment as a necessary criterion in determining civil commitment status. SVP acts have been found to address treatment needs rather than to serve as supplemental punishment to criminal sanctions. SVP statutes require a mental abnormality to be found, in addition to the showing of dangerousness.

5. **C**

In *Washington v. Harper*, Mr. Harper was a prisoner at a state institution for convicted felons with serious mental illness. He refused medications, and the state institution followed its policy of a hospital committee review of the need for medications over objection. Mr. Harper filed suit, claiming that a judicial hearing with findings of substituted judgment was necessary. The U.S. Supreme Court ruled that the hospital review and using professional judgment regarding medications satisfied due process.

6. **C**

In *Robinson v. California*, the U.S. Supreme Court ruled that people addicted to drugs could not be criminally punished for the "status" of being addicted (therefore A, B, and D are false). They could, however, be mandated to treatment in the interests of public health and regulating drug trafficking (therefore E is false). This allowed laws specifically addressing addicted people differently than nonaddicted people, though only under strict limitations.

7. **A**

The U.S. Supreme Court has considered "currently prevailing standards of decency" that "mark the progress of a maturing society" and as a result ruled against precedent set in prior cases. The *Roper v. Simmons* ruling went against precedent set in *Stanford v. Kentucky* and found that execution of juvenile offenders was a violation of the Eighth Amendment based on evidence that American society's opinion had evolved. The *Payne v. Tennessee* ruling did go against precedent set in *Booth v. Maryland*. However, this decision was not based on the evolution of America's opinion but rather the opinion of the court that the *Booth* decision had been "badly reasoned" and that stare decisis (common law concept that precedent is binding) was not an "inexorable command." The *Ford v. Wainwright* decision cited a long-standing "ancestral legacy" in common law that stands against executing the insane.

8. **E**

The U.S. Supreme Court did not opine about the substantive or procedural issues in the case. Rather, the focus was on whether Congress had the power to enact the federal statute that allowed for civil commitment of a sex offender after completion of his sentence. The Court had previously addressed issues of double jeopardy and equal protection as well as ex post facto and procedural standards in its opinions on state statutes, such as in *Kansas v. Hendricks*.

9. **D**

The accused in a federal prosecution must prove incompetence by a "preponderance of the evidence" (more likely than not). *Cooper v. Oklahoma* held that an Oklahoma law proving a defendant's incompetence by "clear and convincing evidence" violates due process by allowing the state to put a defendant on trial who is more likely than not incompetent. The standard of "beyond a reasonable doubt" (used in criminal matters) is a higher standard than "clear and convincing evidence" and thus would make it even more likely that incompetent defendants are put on trial. "Without due cause" is not a recognized standard.

10. **D**

In *People v. Patterson*, the New York Court of Appeals held that the state can place the burden of proving EED on the defendant without violating the defendant's constitutional due process protections. In EED cases, which are never civil in nature, the distress is not necessarily presumed and has nothing to do with insanity considerations.

11. **D**

In *Miranda*, the suspect did indeed sign a confession in which he stated that he knew of his rights and that his statement may be used against him—but only after he had been in custody for several hours. Therefore, the case was overturned not because he did not know his rights but because having been in custody for several hours, he might have felt coerced to confess even though the police may not have committed any particular misconduct. The remaining answers were not cited in this or any other case. Subsequent to *Miranda*, Congress passed a statute that appeared to return the standard for judging the admissibility of confessions to one of a "totality of circumstances." However, the *Miranda* decision survived several challenges, as recently as 2004, and the so-called *Miranda* warning remains a continuing requirement.

12. **D**

The U.S. Supreme Court ruled in *Estelle v. Smith* that a defendant's Fifth Amendment right against self-incrimination and Sixth Amendment right to counsel had been violated when a psychiatrist conducted a competency to stand trial evaluation and later used information obtained at a sentencing hearing. The Court reasoned that his Fifth Amendment right was violated because he was not aware that he could refuse and that the information he provided could be used against him. The Court also reasoned that because there had been no notice to defense counsel, he did not have the opportunity to consult his counsel about whether or not he should participate.

13. **A**

The attempted assassination of Ronald Reagan by John Hinckley and the ensuing insanity defense trial prompted the Insanity Defense Reform Act of 1984, in which the burden of proof in federal courts shifted from the prosecution having to prove a defendant's sanity beyond a reasonable doubt to the defendant having to prove insanity by clear and convincing evidence.

14. **A**

Drope v. Missouri held that competency should be considered at any time where sufficient doubt arises about a defendant's current competence in an effort to protect the defendant's right to a fair trial, which includes protection of his or her due process.

15. **C**

This question has been addressed in the context of both prison-based treatment and postincarceration SVP programs. *McKune v. Lile*, 536 U.S. 24 (2002) concerns treatment during incarceration, with the finding that the Fifth Amendment is not violated by a prison clinical rehabilitation program with a legitimate penological objective if the consequences of refusal to participate are related to the program objective and are not significant hardships relative to the prison environment. *Allen v. Illinois*, 478 U.S. 364 (1986), found that due process did not require Fifth Amendment protections against self-incrimination in SVP acts.

16. **D**

In *Montana v. Egelhoff*, the U.S. Supreme Court affirmed that state law was not required by due process to allow entry of evidence of voluntary intoxication in criminal cases. It based this decision on the fact that common law had not universally acknowledged voluntary intoxication as a mitigating factor. Citing examples such as hearsay, the Court went on to discuss how various classes of potential evidence are routinely excluded. The *Egelhoff* decision had nothing to do with the insanity defense, which is not available in all states.

17. **C**

The American Medical Association (AMA) states that physicians may not participate in executions. The AMA also states that testifying to competency to stand trial, testifying to relevant medical evidence during trial, or testifying to medical aspects of aggravating or mitigating circumstances during the penalty phase of a capital case does *not* constitute physician participation in an execution. The AMA Principles of Medical Ethics, with Annotations Especially Applicable to Psychiatry, state that a psychiatrist should not participate in a legally authorized execution. Neither the APA nor the American Academy of Psychiatry and the Law (AAPL) prohibits psychiatrists from providing treatment to patients who are incompetent to be executed, although the AMA recommends that no psychiatrist treat an inmate solely for the purpose of restoring competence to be executed. The AAPL does not prohibit psychiatrists from conducting competency to be sentenced evaluations.

Please see the relevant ethical guidelines:
1AMA—http://www.ama-assn.org/ama/pub/physician-resources/
    medical-ethics/code-medical-ethics.page
APA—http://www.psych.org/practice/ethics
AAPL—http://www.aapl.org/ethics.htm

18. **A**

Voluntary and knowing. In *Miranda*, the Supreme Court determined that in order for a confession to be voluntary and knowing, the suspect who confessed had to have been apprised of his rights by the police. Informed consent is the standard for agreeing to medical procedures, established in, among other cases, *Natanson v. Kline.* Clear and convincing is a level of proof found in some civil cases where significant liberty interests are at stake, such as civil commitment and right to refuse treatment. Competence and intelligence are general terms that may be included in particular standards for decision making in civil and criminal matters.

19. **C**

Dusky v. U.S. first established that the test for competency to stand trial should be "whether he has sufficient present ability to consult with his lawyer with a reasonable degree of rational understanding—and whether he has a rational as well as factual understanding of the proceedings against him." *Drope v. Missouri* held that competency to stand trial should be considered at any time during a trial where sufficient doubt as to the defendant's competency arises. *Jackson v. Indiana* held that indefinite commitment due to incompetency to stand trial was a violation of the Equal Protection Clause and Due Process Clauses of the Fourteenth Amendment. *Wilson v. U.S.* held that amnesia does not make defendants incompetent as long as they are able to assist their attorney, can testify on their own behalf, and can extrinsically reconstruct the evidence in light of their amnesia.

20. **D**

Ake v. Oklahoma found that a state's denial of an indigent, capital defendant's access to a psychiatric consultant if he or she is pursuing an insanity defense violates the Fourteenth Amendment's due process guarantee.

21. **C**

In *Ibn-Tamas v. U.S.*, the DC Court of Appeals reversed the trial court's decision in excluding expert testimony regarding the "battered wife syndrome." The court found that the expert's statements were beyond the knowledge of the ordinary jury and that the expert testimony likely had more probative value than prejudicial effect. The court did not opine on the legitimacy of the "battered wife syndrome" and in fact returned the case to the trial court to determine the legitimacy of the expert's credentials and of the syndrome in question. Both psychiatrists as well as psychologists can be expert in trauma-related reactions, and there is no blanket protection for retaliatory violence against one's abusers.

22. **E**

The courts in Does #1–5 and Millard were concerned about the punitive aspects related to being a registered sex offender. In both cases, the courts detailed the loss of freedoms which hampered reintegration into society. In Does #1–5, the court reasoned that such a loss could, theoretically, be justified by a state interest in public safety, but the court did not find evidence of enhanced safety. In both Does #1–5 and Millard, the sexual offender registration acts were seen as disproportionate and unjustified continued punishment, and therefore unconstitutional.

23. **C**

The Prison Litigation Reform Act (PLRA) of 1995 is a congressional statute designed to regulate and limit the number of cases filed by prisoners. In the 2011 Supreme Court case of *Brown v. Plata*, the State of California challenged the authority of a three-judge district court to order the reduction of the state prison population as a measure to improve deteriorating medical and mental health care for prisoners. The Supreme Court held that the lower court's decision was allowed under the PLRA.

24. **D**

A diminished capacity defense is not constitutionally required by due process (neither is a not guilty by reason of insanity plea) but is intimately concerned with a defendant's criminal state of mind and intent in the criminal act. Diminished capacity defenses originate from the defense but must be done so by a competent defendant. The benefit of using this defense is for mitigation, not acquittal (as in NGRI defenses).

25. **A**

SVP commitment proceedings have been found to be civil proceedings due to the goal of treatment rather than punishment. Therefore, the courts have ruled that due process requires that there be a finding of mental disorder, though the term can be defined in various ways, including by terms such as "mental illness" or "mental abnormality," and personality disorder may be considered. As with other forms of civil commitment hearings, the mental disorder in question must have a relationship with the individual's risk of dangerousness, in this case committing sexual offenses.

26. **B**
Prison officials may be held liable for deliberate indifference only if they are aware of a "substantial risk of serious harm" and they "disregard that risk by failing to take reasonable measures to abate it." The 1994 Supreme Court case of *Farmer v. Brennan* involved a suit brought by a male-to-female transsexual who alleged a violation of her Eighth Amendment rights by prison officials after she was beaten and raped by another inmate in a federal penitentiary.

27. **E**
Ford v. Wainwright (1986) addressed the issue of a mentally ill person's competence to be executed and held that the Eighth Amendment prohibited the execution of the insane. *Atkins v. Virginia* (2002) found that execution of the mentally retarded was barred by the Eighth Amendment. *Roper v. Simmons* (2005) similarly found that it was unconstitutional to subject offenders who were under the age of 18 at the time of committing a capital offense to the death penalty. *Estelle v. Smith* (1981) dealt with the use of psychiatric testimony to predict future dangerousness. In *State v. Perry* (1992), the Louisiana Supreme Court addressed the question whether the state could give antipsychotic medication involuntarily to an incompetent death row inmate to make him competent to be executed.

28. **E**
State v. Perry was a Louisiana Supreme Court case that determined that involuntary medication administered merely for the purpose of restoring competency for execution is an unjustified invasion of privacy and added a degrading indignity to the punishment that was cruel and excessive. In *Washington v. Harper*, the court considered whether a prisoner is entitled to a judicial hearing when seeking to refuse psychiatric medication and found that due process requires liberty interests to be balanced against the prisoner's medical interest and the state's interest in prison safety.

29. **B**
In this case, Mr. Connelly had provided a full confession to murder while affected by command auditory hallucinations. The police taking the confession were not coercive in any way, but the confession was clearly not the result of a "rational intellect and free will." The Court held that police coercion was the determinative factor in deciding whether a confession should be suppressed. In the case, *Miranda* rights were clearly presented in a timely fashion. Illegal search and seizure are not relevant considerations to the appropriateness of a confession.

31. **B**

Vitek v. Jones was a 1980 U.S. Supreme Court case in which a Nebraska prisoner challenged the authority of the state to transfer him to a psychiatric hospital in violation of the Due Process Clause of the Fourteenth Amendment. The Court ruled that the transfer of a prisoner to a mental hospital has stigmatizing consequences beyond those imposed by incarceration and exposed Mr. Jones to treatment over his objection.

32. **E**

The legal holding in *Connelly* pertains to the constitutional guarantee on due process of law, specifically that coercive police behavior is required to invalidate a confession. This protection is codified in the Fourteenth Amendment. The First Amendment protects freedom of speech, religion, and the press. The Second Amendment protects the right to bear arms. The Fourth Amendment prohibits unlawful search and seizure. The Eighth Amendment prohibits cruel and unusual punishment.

33. **C**

In *Atkins v. Virginia*, the majority held that imposing the death penalty on the mentally retarded would not measurably contribute to the goals of retribution or deterrence. They reasoned that the deficiencies of mentally retarded offenders diminish their personal culpability such that the most extreme form of punishment is not warranted and that their cognitive and behavioral impairments made it unlikely that they would control their conduct based on knowledge of the possibility of the death penalty. The Court also considered that mentally retarded offenders are less able to meaningfully assist in their defense and as a result have an increased risk of wrongful execution. The Court also took into account the large number of states that prohibited the execution of the mentally retarded and polling data that showed consensus among Americans that executing the mentally retarded is wrong. Mental retardation in and of itself does not necessarily render an offender incompetent.

34. **D**

The presence of mental disorder alone is not sufficient to find lack of control. The ruling in *Kansas v. Crane*, 534 U.S. 407 (2002), discussed the lack of "mathematical precision" possible in determining lack of control, in part because the distinction between "emotional" and "volitional" is not always clear. Complete lack of control over behavior is not necessary; proof of serious difficulty is adequate.

35. **C**

Wilson v. U.S., a case heard in the U.S. Court of Appeals, D.C. Circuit, held that amnesia did not make a defendant incompetent if available ancillary information was available to construct knowledge of an event in order to mount a defense. It also held that such defendants should be able to follow the proceedings against them, discuss them rationally with their attorney, and testify on their own behalf.

36. **B**

Under the Eighth Amendment, prison officials may be held liable if they are aware of a "substantial risk of serious harm" and they "disregard that risk by failing to take reasonable measures to abate it." The 1994 U.S. Supreme Court case of *Farmer v. Brennan* involved a suit brought by a male-to-female transsexual who alleged a violation of her Eighth Amendment rights by prison officials after she was beaten and raped by a male inmate in a federal penitentiary. The test applied to this case was that of "subjective recklessness."

37. **A**

In *Payne v. Tennessee*, the U.S. Supreme Court reconsidered its prior position in the *Booth* and *Gathers* decisions. The Court determined that victim impact statements should be allowed to aid a jury in understanding the "uniqueness" of the victim as an individual and in assessing the degree of harm caused by the crime, which is directly related to the defendant's moral culpability. The state should also be afforded the opportunity to rebut mitigating evidence presented by the defense at sentencing. It is possible that psychiatrists could be asked to testify about the psychological impact of the crime on the victim's family.

38. **B**

In this case the defendant presents with the cognitive difficulties required of *M'Naghten*. In the other scenarios the defendants' ability to control their actions may be in question, but they may all be aware of what they are doing or that what they are doing is wrong.

39. **E**

The "necessary and proper" clause is found in Article I of the Constitution, which specifies that Congress has the power "to make all law which shall be necessary and proper for carrying into execution the foregoing powers and all other powers vested by this Constitution." The First Amendment guarantees the right to free speech and assembly. The Fifth Amendment guarantees the right against self-incrimination. The Eighth Amendment prohibits cruel and unusual punishment. The Fourteenth Amendment guarantees due process and equal protection and is the amendment through which all the amendments are made obligatory on the states as well as the federal government.

40. **B**

An ALI jurisdiction states that a person is not responsible for criminal conduct if at the time of such conduct as a result of mental disease he lacks substantial capacity either to appreciate the wrongfulness of his conduct or to conform his conduct to the requirements of the law. Answer B comes closest to presenting a scenario in which the defendant was not able to appreciate the wrongfulness of his actions or to conform his conduct to the law.

41. E

In *Robinson v. California*, 370 U.S. 660 (1962), the U.S. Supreme Court ruled that it was cruel and unusual punishment to arrest people for a status they could not control, if they had not performed any other antisocial or disorderly behavior. Possible intent to commit a crime in the undefined future is not in itself a prosecutable crime. All the other answer choices are taken directly from the text of the opinion as valid forms of state regulation. The Court ruled that states maintained broad powers to impose criminal sanctions against the unauthorized manufacture, prescription, sale, purchase, or possession of narcotics within their borders. It also ruled that it was not cruel and unusual to impose compulsory treatment for those addicted to narcotics—with periods of involuntary confinement as part of a treatment program—and penal sanctions for a failure to comply with established compulsory treatment procedures. Finally, the Court ruled that other strategies at the disposal of the states could include public health education and efforts to ameliorate the economic and social conditions under which drug abuse flourishes.

42. E

Answers (A) through (D) have all been raised in challenges to sexual offender commitment statutes. Double jeopardy and ex post facto lawmaking were raised by *In re Young and Cunningham*, 857 P.2d 989 (1993), and *Kansas v. Hendricks*, 521 U.S. 346 (1997). Due process issues were raised in *Specht v. Patterson*, 386 U.S. 605 (1967), *In re Young and Cunningham*, and *Kansas v. Hendricks*. The Fifth Amendment was addressed in *Allen v. Illinois*, 478 U.S. 364 (1986), and *McKune v. Lile*, 536 U.S. 24 (2002).

43. A

In supporting New York State's right to place the burden to prove aspects of EED on the defendant, the court of appeals differentiated the state's law from Maine's EED law, which had recently been struck down by the U.S. Supreme Court in *Mullaney v. Wilbur*, 421 U.S. 684 (1975). The New York state law still required the state to prove all elements of the crime and so did not violate due process. The decision in *Patterson* was unrelated to its legislative history and has nothing to do with voluntary intoxication. EED is not based in the U.S. Constitution (being only available in certain states).

44. B

Mr. Powell was decidedly *not* convicted for the "status" of being an alcoholic, as this would have been in direct contradiction of *Robinson v. California*. He was in fact convicted for the "act" of being intoxicated in public; he was not alleged to have committed any other crime, including murder. The Court opinion briefly made reference to the debate regarding responsibility for criminal actions as it related to the insanity defense by mentioning two cases. In one, the U.S. Court of Appeals for the D.C. Circuit decided *Durham v. U.S.* (1954), adopting the "product test" to determine the validity of an insanity defense; it states that "an accused is not criminally responsible if his unlawful act was the product of mental disease or defect." The other, a historic English case, resulted in the *M'Naghten* rule, which stated in summary that insanity was a defense if the party was unable to tell right from wrong at the time of the crime. Other than using these cases as abstract legal analogies, the Court refused to define an insanity defense in constitutional terms and did not opine on their relationship to Mr. Powell's case.

45. **B**
In *Sell v. U.S.*, Dr. Sell was found incompetent to stand trial and, while hospitalized, refused antipsychotic medication. Forced medication was authorized, and Sell appealed. The U.S. Supreme Court ruled that the government is permitted to involuntarily administer antipsychotic medications to certain mentally ill defendants in order to render them competent to stand trial, but the Court outlined necessary procedures, which included that the treatment should be unlikely to have side effects that undermine fairness of a trial, that the recommended treatment should be the least intrusive and medically appropriate, and that the treatment should be necessary to further government trial-related interests.

46. **C**
Indiana v. Edwards held that the Constitution permits states to insist upon counsel for those competent to stand trial under the standard set forth by *Dusky v. U.S.* but incompetent to conduct their own trial proceedings. The Court noted that *Dusky* alone was not sufficient and assumed representation within the standard itself. It also pointed to the variability in mental illness with regard to its course over time and the variability in the way it interferes with a defendant's function. Furthermore, permitting self-representation to a defendant who lacks the capacity to conduct his or her defense without counsel does not "affirm the dignity" of the defendant and does not "appear fair to all who observe them."

47. **E**
For years, the state of California failed to comply with court-ordered remedial efforts to improve the delivery of both medical and mental health care to its prisoners. In 2008, a three-judge district court combined two class action suits (one for medical care, one for mental health care) and ordered to have the prison population reduced to 137.5% of its designed capacity

to rectify overcrowding in California prisons, which was determined to be a primary cause for the poor medical and mental health care.

48. **B**

This question is answered by *McKune v. Lile*, 536 U.S. 24 (2002). The prison program challenged by Lile required him to accept responsibility for the crime of conviction and detail prior sexual activities, including potential uncharged offenses, with refusal to participate leading to consequences of reduction in privileges and possible transfer to a higher-security unit. The Supreme Court decision allows for the program to be incentivized through prison privileges and holds that Fifth Amendment protections against self-incrimination do not prevent treatment programs from requiring participants to disclose sexual histories and prior behaviors. Availability of sex offender treatment during incarceration has been cited as an issue in legislative and mental health community discussions but has not been made a requirement by court decisions.

49. **D**

As established in *Hall v. Florida* and *Moore v. Texas*, the Supreme Court held that considering an IQ number alone created an unacceptable risk that persons with an intellectual disability will be executed in violation of the Eighth and Fourteenth Amendments.

50. **C**

Most clinicians agree that medical testimony should stem from a competent and reliable comprehensive clinical psychiatric risk assessment that is rooted in evidence-based practice standards for medical evaluation and that considers all relevant clinical and historical information, including data from standardized risk assessment tools. Answer "A" is incorrect because predicating future dangerousness is not an exact science. Answer "B" relates to the decision in *Buck v. Davis*, 137 S. Ct. 759, 197 L. Ed. 2d 1 (2017), in which the Supreme Court held that to punish someone based on an immutable characteristic is a disturbing departure from a basic premise of our criminal justice system—that the law punishes people for what they do, not who they are. Answer "D" is a mischaracterization of the link between mental illness and dangerousness. Research shows that the vast majority of people who are violent do not suffer from mental illnesses. The absolute risk of violence among the mentally ill as a group is still shown to be very small.

SECTION VI

Miscellaneous

CHAPTER 29

Immigration

JEREMY COLLEY AND HEATHER ELLIS CUCOLO

PADILLA V. KENTUCKY, 559 U.S. 356 (2010)

Link to case: https://supreme.justia.com/cases/federal/us/559/356/

Question: Does the Sixth Amendment impose an affirmative duty on a criminal defense attorney to advise his client that mandatory deportation will result from a guilty plea?

Answer: Yes.

In this case, Jose Padilla, a permanent U.S. resident, entered a guilty plea to three drug charges on advice from his lawyer. Padilla's attorney believed that the length of time upon which Padilla was in the country would prevent him from being deported. Contrary to that belief, deportation was almost a certain consequence for the type of drug-related conviction that Padilla faced. He subsequently filed for postconviction relief, arguing that he was misadvised about the potential for deportation as a consequence of his guilty plea.

The U.S. Supreme Court held that counsel must inform a client whether his plea carries a risk of deportation. Although deportation is a civil matter, the Court recognized that it is inextricably linked to the decision to plead guilty in a criminal case. John Paul Stevens, writing for the majority, noted that the number of offenses resulting in deportation has grown exponentially and thus, because deportation is virtually certain for many noncitizens convicted of crimes, the importance of accurate advice as to the immigration consequences of a plea has never been more vital. The

Court reasoned that counsel's advice with respect to deportation is not categorically removed from the scope of the Sixth Amendment.

In this case, Mr. Padilla's Sixth Amendment right to counsel was violated because counsel should have known or learned that a guilty plea would make Mr. Padilla eligible for deportation. The Court then remanded the case to the Supreme Court of Kentucky to determine whether Mr. Padilla was prejudiced by his counsel's deficiency. Other states have followed the Supreme Court's holding in *Padilla v. Kentucky* with an emphasis on the state court's role in advising a noncitizen defendant during plea proceeding.

MATTER OF M-A-M, 25 I. & N. DEC. 474, 474 (BIA 2011)

Link to case: https://www.justice.gov/sites/default/files/eoir/legacy/2014/07/25/3711.pdf

Question: Is evidence of lack of competence to participate a relevant consideration in immigration proceedings?

Answer: Yes.

In M-A-M, the Board of Immigration Appeals (BIA) set forth a test for immigration judges to apply to determine where an individual is competent to participate in a removal hearing. Decisive factors were laid out by the BIA to assess the individual's capacity to participate: whether the respondent understands the nature and object of the proceedings; whether the respondent can consult with the attorney or representative (if there is one); and whether the respondent has a reasonable opportunity to examine adverse evidence, present favorable evidence, and cross-examine government witnesses.

As in regular (i.e., non-immigration-based) competency hearings, the respondent is presumed to be competent, and M-A-M only requires an immigration judge to apply the test when the indicia of mental incompetency is raised. Such indicia may derive from observations by the immigration judge or either party of the respondent's functioning and behaviour, or testimonial evidence and/or documentation submitted as part of the record. The BIA instructed immigration judges to consider indicia of incompetency throughout the duration of the removal proceeding. The BIA emphasized that measures needed to assess competency will vary from case to case and might include basic questions to assess the respondent's ability to understand the nature and object of the proceedings, additional time for the parties to collect relevant documentary evidence, an order for a competency evaluation, and/or testimony from family or close friends.

In addition, M-A-M obligates the Department of Homeland Security (DHS) to provide the court with any evidence in its possession bearing on the respondent's mental competency (DHS is required to produce documents bearing only on a respondent's competency). Once the full assessment is completed, the immigration judge must articulate on the record his or her reasoning and decision regarding the respondent's competency. Should a respondent not be sufficiently competent to proceed with a hearing, the judge has discretion to apply appropriate safeguards. The BIA listed available safeguards as examples, but noted that the list was not exhaustive: legal representation (in immigration hearings, right to counsel is not guaranteed); identification of someone to assist the respondent and/or his or her legal representative; appointment of a guardian; opportunity to restore competency; closing the hearing to the public; waiving respondent's appearance at the hearing; and reserving the right to appeal. If a fair hearing cannot be assured by the available procedural safeguards, M-A-M permits an indefinite stay of proceedings pending the exploration of other options such as treatment.

CHAPTER 30

Gun Ownership

JEREMY COLLEY AND HEATHER ELLIS CUCOLO

DISTRICT OF COLUMBIA V. HELLER, 554 U.S. 570 (2008)

Link to case: https://supreme.justia.com/cases/federal/us/554/570/

Question: Did the District of Columbia's total prohibition of the possession of handguns violate the Second Amendment?

Answer: Yes.

Dick Heller was a police officer in Washington, D.C., who attempted to register a handgun, which he intended to keep in his home. The District of Columbia refused his application, citing local law that banned registration of handguns, for any purpose. Heller brought a claim to the Federal District Court for the District of Columbia that the law violated his Second Amendment right to bear firearms. The District Court initially dismissed the claim, arguing Heller did not have standing. Heller appealed, and ultimately the U.S. Supreme Court granted certiorari.

Justice Scalia penned the majority opinion, establishing via an analysis of the meaning of the Second Amendment at the time it was written, as well as its interpretation by the courts since then, that it establishes the right of an individual to bear arms whether or not he or she participates in a militia, as long as the use of such weapons is for a lawful purpose, such as self-defense. That said, the Court was clear that this right is not absolute: "Although we do not undertake an exhaustive historical analysis today of the full scope of the Second Amendment, nothing in our opinion should be taken to cast doubt on longstanding prohibitions on the possession of firearms by felons and the mentally ill, or laws forbidding the carrying of firearms in sensitive places such as schools and government buildings, or laws imposing conditions and qualifications on the commercial sale of arms."

Justices Stevens and Justice Breyer filed separate dissents; Stevens, relying on the prior U.S. Supreme Court decision in *United States v. Miller*, 307 U.S. 174 (1939), did not dispute that the Second Amendment established a right of a state militia to bear arms, but maintained that it does not circumscribe the right of the state to limit individual gun ownership. Justice Breyer agreed with Steven's analysis, but goes further to elaborate that the state interest in combating gun violence via regulation of gun ownership is a compelling one.

MCDONALD V. CITY OF CHICAGO, 561 U.S. 742 (2010)

Link to case: https://supreme.justia.com/cases/federal/us/561/742/

Question: Does the Second Amendment, via the Fourteenth, apply to the states, in order to protect a citizen's right to bear firearms for lawful purposes?

Answer: Yes.

Otis McDonald, Adam Orlov, Colleen Lawson, and David Lawson, all residents of Chicago, as well as the National Rifle Association, filed lawsuits in the U.S. District Court for the Northern District of Illinois, claiming that Chicago's ban on individual ownership of handguns violated their Second Amendment rights, guaranteed to state citizens via the Fourteenth Amendment, in the wake of the Court's decision 2 years prior in *District of Columbia v. Heller*, 554 U.S. 570 (2008). The District Court, and the Court of Appeals for the Seventh Circuit, both dismissed the claim, upholding Chicago's ban on handgun ownership. The U.S. Supreme Court granted certiorari.

Justice Alito authored the majority opinion, and he held that the Second Amendment did indeed apply to individual citizens of states. Although the *Heller* decision had addressed its meaning in the District of Columbia only, the majority held that Chicago's handgun prohibition was also unconstitutional, writing "it is clear that the Framers and ratifiers of the Fourteenth Amendment counted the right to keep and bear arms among those fundamental rights necessary to our system of ordered liberty."

The dissenting opinions, by Justices Stevens and Breyer as in *Heller*, phrased the question as follows: "The question we must decide is whether the interest in keeping in the home a firearm of one's choosing—a handgun, for petitioners—is one that is 'comprised within the term liberty' in the

Fourteenth Amendment," as only rights that are so comprised apply to state citizens. Neither firearm ownership, nor self-defense, falls within that definition, Stevens wrote.

TYLER V. HILLSDALE COUNTY SHERIFF'S DEPARTMENT, 837 F.3D 678 (6TH CIR. 2016)

Question: Does the Second Amendment forbid Congress from permanently prohibiting firearm possession by currently healthy individuals who were previously civilly committed to a psychiatric hospital?

Answer: Maybe.

Mr. Clifford Tyler was committed to a psychiatric hospital in Michigan in 1986, when he was 44 years old. At the time, he and his wife were divorcing, after Tyler's wife left him for another man and took off with a substantial sum of money. In this context, Tyler became depressed; after seeing him hitting himself in the head, Tyler's daughters sought to have him admitted to the Ypsilanti Regional Center for management of his suicide risk. He was hospitalized for 4 weeks, refused medication, and did not seek treatment after discharge. He returned to work and remarried in 1999. In 2011, he attempted to purchase a firearm in Hillsdale County, Michigan, but was unable to do so, via 18 U.S.C. § 922(g)(4), which prohibits individuals previously committed to a psychiatric facility from buying guns. Moreover, neither Michigan nor the Federal Bureau of Alcohol, Tobacco and Firearms (ATF)—because of budget cuts—was able to evaluate whether Tyler's eligibility could be restored; neither could conduct an examination to determine if Tyler remained mentally ill and dangerous. Tyler sued, claiming that what amounted to a lifetime ban on his ability to own firearms stemming from his civil commitment 30 years prior violated his Second Amendment right to bear arms.

Tyler's claim was dismissed by the federal district court for failure to state a claim, arguing that federal law allowed restriction of firearms from certain groups, including the mentally ill, citing the U.S. Supreme Court decisions in *Heller* and *McDonald*. Tyler appealed, and the Court of Appeals heard the case twice, referred to as *Tyler I* (2014) and *Tyler II* (2016). In *Tyler I*, the court determined that § 922(g)(4) was not inherently immune from constitutional scrutiny, and, in fact, that to abridge a citizen's Second Amendment right, a law must withstand strict scrutiny, given its fundamental nature. *Tyler II* superseded *Tyler I*, as the court considered the particular facts of Mr. Tyler's claim and determined that intermediate rather than strict scrutiny was appropriate and that the state had failed to demonstrate how a permanent ban on Tyler's right to bear arms based on his distant civil commitment alone was reasonably related to compelling state interests of reducing crime and preventing suicide. The court, in reversing and remanding to the district court, offered two options under which § 922(g)(4) could be applied constitutionally—the state could show that a single past civil commitment did elevate an individual's lifelong risk so as to justify an ongoing ownership ban, or the state could reassess the risk of those in Mr. Tyler's situation and provide an avenue to restore their Second Amendment rights.

WOLLSCHLAEGER V. GOVERNOR OF FLORIDA, 760 F. 3D 1195 (2017)

Link to case: https://www.leagle.com/decision/infco20140728107

Question: Does Florida's ban on doctors' discussing the risks of gun ownership with patients violate the doctors' First Amendment right to free speech?

Answer: No.

Florida's Firearm Owner's Privacy Act, which went into effect in 2011, made it illegal for physicians to make a "verbal or written inquiry" about a patient's gun ownership unless the physician "in good faith" believed that doing so was "relevant to the patient's medical care or safety, or the safety of others." In response, a number of Florida physicians filed a lawsuit, claiming that the law violated their right to free speech guaranteed by the First Amendment, applied to state citizens via the Fourteenth Amendment. The District Court found in favor of the physicians, but the state appealed, arguing that the law regulated professional practice, not speech, and, therefore, the physicians did not have a constitutional claim.

In 2014, the Court of Appeals reversed, via a three judge panel, finding in favor of the state, arguing that the law promoted several compelling state interests which needed to be weighed against the circumscription of a physician's communications, bearing in mind the inherent power imbalance in the doctor–patient relationship. These compelling state interests included a patient's right to privacy, and by extension, a patient's right to bear arms via the Second Amendment and to receive proper medical care without fear of harassment or discrimination because of owning a gun. The court found that the limitation on speech was "incidental" and did not extent outside of the examination room.

The dissent maintained that the state interests enumerated by the majority must be weighed not only again a physician's right to speech, but also to the potential harm patients may suffer as a result. Thus, a physician's inquiry about firearms is certainly "relevant to the patient's medical care," as defined in the law: "difficulties arise because Appellees and the State have different definitions of 'relevant.' Many doctors and medical organizations assert that it is always relevant to ask about—and thus, to record—firearm-ownership information. . . Doctors thus quite legitimately insist that asking firearm-related questions as a matter of course and recording the information in medical files is good for their patients' health and for the public's safety."

In 2017, the physicians appealed for a hearing en banc; the 11th Circuit ruled 10-1 in favor of the physicians, arguing along the lines of the dissent in the 2014 decision that Florida law did encroach upon physician's right to free speech.

CHAPTER 31

Questions on Immigration and Gun Ownership

QUESTIONS

1. The right to bear what kind of "arms," as it appears in the Second Amendment, was the primary focus of *District of Columbia v. Heller*?
   A. Rifles
   B. Shotguns
   C. Handguns
   D. Machine guns
   E. Bump stocks

2. What key constitutional question distinguished *District of Columbia v. Heller* from *McDonald v. City of Chicago*?
   A. How many handguns can a citizen own?
   B. Is the possession of grenades protected by the Second Amendment?
   C. Does the Second Amendment apply to the states, via the Fourteenth Amendment?
   D. Can a state mandate gun safety training prior to issuing a handgun permit?
   E. Can a state revoke a citizen's lawfully possessed handgun for having too many parking tickets?

3. Can a state restrict a citizen from possessing firearms because of a history of having been psychiatrically hospitalized against his will?
   A. No, the right to bear arms may not be abridged under any circumstances.
   B. Yes, but only if the citizen was hospitalized because he was dangerous to others.

C. Yes, but only if the citizen used a firearm in a suicide attempt that led to hospitalization.
D. No, but the state can force a patient to take antipsychotics if he wants to regain his right to bear arms.
E. Yes, but the nature and duration of restriction of the citizen's right to bear arms must be reasonably related to a compelling state interest, such as public safety.

ANSWERS

1. **C**

At the time, the District of Columbia prohibited the possession of handguns, even within a resident's home. It did allow residents to own shotguns and rifles, but required that they be unloaded and disassembled or bound by a trigger lock. Heller, in the brining the case, argued that handguns were a vital means of self-defense, and Justice Scalia, in his majority opinion, coupled one's right to be safe in their home to the rights guaranteed via the Second Amendment.

2. **C**

District of Columbia v. Heller established the right to bear arms within its borders; it did not establish whether the Second Amendment—which applied to D.C. given it is Federal territory—applied to the states via the Fourteenth Amendment. *McDonald v. City of Chicago* established that indeed it did apply to the states.

3. **E**

Tyler v. Hillsdale County Sheriff's Department, the court reversed and remanded a lower court decision, and therefore offered no ruling, per se, but in dicta suggested that a state can abridge one's right to bear arms in light of a compelling state interest to do so. Using this rationale, not allowing people civilly committed to a psychiatric hospital to own firearms could be justified, in the name of public safety. However, the court indicated that such a ban, if permanent and absolute, would likely be unconstitutional, unless the state could prove the person seeking to restore his rights continues to pose a risk to the community.

APPENDIX A

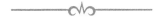

The Bill of Rights and Fourteenth Amendment, U.S. Constitution

Amendments I–X Ratified December 15, 1791; XIV ratified July 9, 1868
Source: www.archives.gov
The Preamble to the Bill of Rights
Congress of the United States
begun and held at the City of New-York, on
Wednesday the fourth of March, one thousand seven hundred and eighty nine.

THE Conventions of a number of the States, having at the time of their adopting the Constitution, expressed a desire, in order to prevent misconstruction or abuse of its powers, that further declaratory and restrictive clauses should be added: And as extending the ground of public confidence in the Government, will best ensure the beneficent ends of its institution.

RESOLVED by the Senate and House of Representatives of the United States of America, in Congress assembled, two thirds of both Houses concurring, that the following Articles be proposed to the Legislatures of the several States, as amendments to the Constitution of the United States, all, or any of which Articles, when ratified by three fourths of the said Legislatures, to be valid to all intents and purposes, as part of the said Constitution; viz.

ARTICLES in addition to, and Amendment of the Constitution of the United States of America, proposed by Congress, and ratified by the Legislatures of the several States, pursuant to the fifth Article of the original Constitution.

AMENDMENT I

Congress shall make no law respecting an establishment of religion, or prohibiting the free exercise thereof; or abridging the freedom of speech, or of the press; or the right of the people peaceably to assemble, and to petition the Government for a redress of grievances.

AMENDMENT II

A well regulated Militia, being necessary to the security of a free State, the right of the people to keep and bear Arms, shall not be infringed.

AMENDMENT III

No Soldier shall, in time of peace be quartered in any house, without the consent of the Owner, nor in time of war, but in a manner to be prescribed by law.

AMENDMENT IV

The right of the people to be secure in their persons, houses, papers, and effects, against unreasonable searches and seizures, shall not be violated, and no Warrants shall issue, but upon probable cause, supported by Oath or affirmation, and particularly describing the place to be searched, and the persons or things to be seized.

AMENDMENT V

No person shall be held to answer for a capital, or otherwise infamous crime, unless on a presentment or indictment of a Grand Jury, except in cases arising in the land or naval forces, or in the Militia, when in actual service in time of War or public danger; nor shall any person be subject for the same offence to be twice put in jeopardy of life or limb; nor shall be compelled in any criminal case to be a witness against himself, nor be deprived of life, liberty, or property, without due process of law; nor shall private property be taken for public use, without just compensation.

AMENDMENT VI

In all criminal prosecutions, the accused shall enjoy the right to a speedy and public trial, by an impartial jury of the State and district wherein the crime shall have been committed, which district shall have been previously ascertained by law, and to be informed of the nature and cause of the accusation; to be confronted with the witnesses against him; to have compulsory process for obtaining witnesses in his favor, and to have the Assistance of Counsel for his defence.

AMENDMENT VII

In Suits at common law, where the value in controversy shall exceed twenty dollars, the right of trial by jury shall be preserved, and no fact tried by a jury, shall be otherwise re-examined in any Court of the United States, than according to the rules of the common law.

AMENDMENT VIII

Excessive bail shall not be required, nor excessive fines imposed, nor cruel and unusual punishments inflicted.

AMENDMENT IX

The enumeration in the Constitution, of certain rights, shall not be construed to deny or disparage others retained by the people.

AMENDMENT X

The powers not delegated to the United States by the Constitution, nor prohibited by it to the States, are reserved to the States respectively, or to the people.

AMENDMENT XIV

Section 1

All persons born or naturalized in the United States, and subject to the jurisdiction thereof, are citizens of the United States and of the State wherein they reside. No State shall make or enforce any law which shall abridge the privileges or immunities of citizens of the United States; nor shall any State deprive any person of life, liberty, or property, without due process of law; nor deny to any person within its jurisdiction the equal protection of the laws.

Section 2

Representatives shall be apportioned among the several States according to their respective numbers, counting the whole number of persons in each State, excluding Indians not taxed. But when the right to vote at any election for the choice of electors for President and Vice-President of the United States, Representatives in Congress, the Executive and Judicial officers of a State, or the members of the Legislature thereof, is denied to any of the male inhabitants of such State, being twenty-one years of age, and citizens of the United States, or in any way abridged, except for participation in rebellion, or other crime, the basis of representation therein shall be reduced in the proportion which the number of such male citizens shall bear to the whole number of male citizens twenty-one years of age in such State.

Section 3

No person shall be a Senator or Representative in Congress, or elector of President and Vice-President, or hold any office, civil or military, under the United States, or under any State, who, having previously taken an oath, as a member of Congress, or as an officer of the United States, or as a member of any State legislature, or as an executive or judicial officer of any State, to support the Constitution of the United States, shall have engaged in insurrection or rebellion against the same, or given aid or comfort to the enemies thereof. But Congress may by a vote of two-thirds of each House, remove such disability.

Section 4

The validity of the public debt of the United States, authorized by law, including debts incurred for payment of pensions and bounties for services in suppressing insurrection or rebellion, shall not be questioned. But neither the United States nor any State shall assume or pay any debt or obligation incurred in aid of insurrection or rebellion against the United States, or any claim for the loss or emancipation of any slave; but all such debts, obligations and claims shall be held illegal and void.

Section 5

The Congress shall have the power to enforce, by appropriate legislation, the provisions of this article.

APPENDIX B

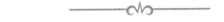

Federal Versus State Jurisdiction and the Supreme Court

In crafting the U.S. Constitution, the intent of the framers was to give limited power to the federal government. Federalism is the fundamental idea that government power is divided between one national government and other, smaller state or regional governments. The founders of the United States wanted the states to have wide discretion to enact laws that are specific to the needs of its individual region and populace. Such laws would be upheld so long as they did not infringe on the Constitution of the United States. In furtherance of this federalism objective, our court system was designed so that state courts had broad oversight and control over the laws that were enacted by their state legislature. The federal courts were thus given limited review power in many of the disputes that govern our daily lives within our individual states. Generally, state and federal court systems do not overlap, and it is only under very specific circumstances that a case in state court can be appealed to a federal court or heard under a right of federal jurisdiction. The most common example manifested in the landmark cases reviewed in this text is when a state case raises a U.S. Constitutional issue (such as equal protection or free speech) or when state law potentially runs afoul of a civil rights statute passed by the U.S. Congress. The ultimate decision-making court in the federal system for such matters is the U.S. Supreme Court.

JURISDICTION OF THE COURTS: STATE VERSUS FEDERAL

Jurisdiction relates to the authority of a particular court to hear a legal case. There are three types of jurisdiction that every state and federal court must possess in order to hear a case. The first is *territorial jurisdiction*, which means that the court has to be in a geographical area over which the law gives that court authority, such as a state. The second is *personal jurisdiction*, which is the authority that a specific court has over a person who is involved in the controversy. Finally, the third is *subject matter jurisdiction*, which relates to whether the court has authority over the subject matter or controversy.

STATE COURTS: GENERAL JURISDICTION

State courts have what is known as *general jurisdiction*, which means that they have the authority to interpret the state laws in which the court sits. For instance, state courts will have jurisdiction over cases that involve crimes committed in violation of state law, such as burglary, assault, battery, murder, and many drug-related crimes. State courts will also have jurisdiction in cases where the state or municipality is a party, such as a state tax violation. Generally, cases that involve juvenile justice, personal injury, real estate, contract disputes, family, divorce and custody, and probate and inheritance are state court general jurisdiction cases.

FEDERAL COURTS: LIMITED JURISDICTION

Federal courts are courts of *limited jurisdiction*, which means that they can only hear certain types of cases. In order for a federal court to hear a state case and exercise its jurisdiction, the case must either raise a *federal question* and/or involve *diversity jurisdiction*.

Federal questions are often used as a basis for removing a case from state courts to federal courts. A federal question allows a federal court to gain *subject-matter jurisdiction* over what would otherwise be a state jurisdiction case. A federal question occurs when the matter in dispute is based on subjects enumerated in the U.S. Constitution or when a federal statute or treaty is involved in the controversy. A federal question might also be raised when a dispute arises from controversies between two or more states, or between the United States and foreign governments. For instance, if a crime violates federal law, such as bank robbery, or involves interstate criminal activity, such as illegal interstate transfer of firearms or kidnapping that takes place across state lines, then the federal court would gain *subject-matter jurisdiction*. Another way a federal question could be raised is when a civil case is based on a federal law such as the Americans with Disabilities Act or antitrust laws that regulate securities trading. All bankruptcy, patent, copyright, Native American, and maritime cases are considered to be federal questions and are heard in the federal courts.

The second way that a federal court can hear a state case is through diversity jurisdiction. Diversity jurisdiction exists only when the amount in controversy is over $75,000 and there is complete *diversity of citizenship* between the parties. For example, diversity jurisdiction exists when a citizen of New York is suing a citizen of California and claiming $76,000 in damages. If the case involves more than two parties, there cannot be citizens of the same state on different side of the litigation; thus, complete diversity is required. For example, diversity jurisdiction exists if a New York citizen sues two citizens, one from California and one from Texas, in the same suit, but it does not exist if the New York citizen is suing a California citizen and another New York citizen.

Without either a *federal question* or *diversity jurisdiction*, the case would remain in the jurisdiction of the state courts.

APPENDIX C

U.S. Federal District Courts

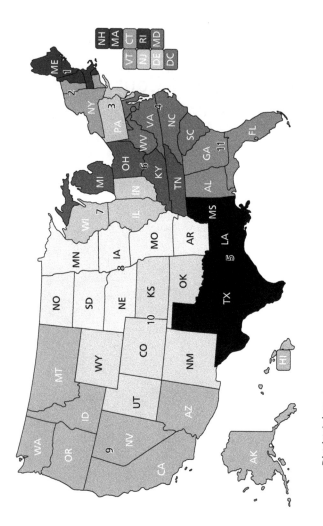

District 1: brown
District 2: yellow
District 3: light pink
District 4: green
District 5: blue
District 6: purple
District 7: pink
District 8: light blue
District 9: orange
District 10: light green
District 11: magenta

APPENDIX D

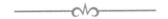

Glossary of Terms

Affirmed: Meaning generally that the higher court has concluded that the lower court decision is correct and will stand as rendered by the lower court. https://www.uscourts.gov/glossary

Appeal: A request made after a trial by a party that has lost on one or more issues that a higher court review the decision to determine if it was correct. To make such a request is "to appeal" or "to take an appeal." One who appeals is called the "appellant"; the other party is the "appellee." https://www.uscourts.gov/glossary

Beyond a reasonable doubt: Standard of proof for all criminal cases and some civil cases such as civil commitment in certain jurisdictions. Sometimes referred to as "to a moral certainty."

Burden of proof: The duty to prove disputed facts. In civil cases, a plaintiff generally has the burden of proving his or her case. In criminal cases, the government has the burden of proving the defendant's guilt. https://www.uscourts.gov/glossary

Certiorari: An order of a higher court to a lower court to send all the documents in a case to it so the higher court can review the lower court's decision. See also *Writ of certiorari*.

Clear and convincing: An evidentiary standard (burden of proof) that means that the evidence is highly and substantially more likely to be true than untrue; the fact finder must be convinced that the contention is highly probable.

Common law: Generally uncodified—meaning that there is no comprehensive compilation of legal rules and statutes. Common law does rely on some scattered statutes, but it is largely based on precedent, meaning the judicial decisions that have already been made in similar cases.

Contempt: Individuals may be cited for contempt when they disobey an order, fail to comply with a request, tamper with documents, withhold evidence, interrupt proceedings through their actions or words, or otherwise defy a public authority or hold it up to ridicule and disrespect.

Declaratory judgment: A judge's statement about someone's rights. For example, a plaintiff may seek a declaratory judgment that a particular statute, as written, violates some constitutional right. https://www.uscourts.gov/glossary

Deterrence: The crime prevention effects of the threat of punishment. Based on a theory of choice in which individuals balance the benefits and costs of crime.

Double jeopardy: The Double Jeopardy Clause in the Fifth Amendment to the U.S. Constitution prohibits anyone from being prosecuted twice for substantially the same crime. The relevant part of the Fifth Amendment states, "No person shall . . . be subject for the same offense to be twice put in jeopardy of life or limb . . . ."

Due process: In criminal law, the constitutional guarantee that a defendant will receive a fair and impartial trial. In civil law, the legal rights of someone who confronts an adverse action threatening liberty or property. https://www.uscourts.gov/glossary

Equal protection: Refers to the idea that a governmental body may not deny people equal protection of its governing laws. The governing body state must treat an individual in the same manner as others in similar conditions and circumstances.

Ex post facto: Forbade by the Constitution of the United States, ex post facto is a law that retroactively makes criminal conduct that was not criminal when performed, increases the punishment for crimes already committed, or changes the rules of procedure in force at the time an alleged crime was committed in a way that is substantially disadvantageous to the accused.

Felony: A serious crime, usually punishable by at least 1 year in prison.

Grand jury: A body of 16–23 citizens who listen to evidence of criminal allegations, which is presented by the prosecutors, and determine whether there is probable cause to believe an individual committed an offense. See also *indictment* and *U.S. attorney.* https://www.uscourts.gov/glossary

Guardian ad litem: An individual who is appointed by a court to protect the interests of a minor or incompetent in a particular matter. State law and local court rules govern the appointment of guardian ad litems.

Judicial gatekeeping: For the purposes of this text, judicial gatekeeping was derived from the case *Daubert v. Merrell Dow Pharmaceuticals.* The decision in *Daubert* illuminated and heightened the crucial role of the judiciary as the gatekeeper for scientific testimony in the courtroom.

Misdemeanor: An offense punishable by 1 year of imprisonment or less.

Moot: Not subject to a court ruling because the controversy has not actually arisen, or it has ended. https://www.uscourts.gov/glossary

Notice: Information, usually in writing in all legal proceedings, of all documents filed, decisions, requests, motions, petitions, and upcoming dates. Notice is a vital principle of fairness and due process in legal procedure and must be given to both parties, to all those affected by a lawsuit or legal proceeding, to the opposing attorney, and to the court.

Per curiuam opinion: Latin, meaning "for the court." In appellate courts, often refers to an unsigned opinion. https://www.uscourts.gov/glossary

Postconviction relief: A general term related to appeals of criminal convictions, which may include release, new trial, modification of sentence, and such other relief as may be proper and just. The court may also make supplementary orders to the relief granted, concerning such matters as rearraignment, retrial, custody, and release.

Precedent: A court decision in an earlier case with facts and legal issues similar to a dispute currently before a court. Judges will generally "follow precedent"—meaning that they use the principles established in earlier cases to decide new cases that have similar facts and raise similar legal issues. A judge will disregard precedent if a party can show that the earlier case was wrongly decided, or that it differed in some significant way from the current case. https://www.uscourts.gov/glossary

Preponderance of the evidence: This is the burden of proof in a civil trial. An evidentiary standard used in a burden of proof analysis that is met when the party with the burden convinces the fact finder that there is a greater than 50% chance that the claim is true.

Privilege: A special and exclusive legal advantage, allowance, permission, or right such as a benefit, exemption, power, or immunity.

Procedural due process: Procedural due process refers to the constitutional requirement that when the federal government acts in such a way that denies a citizen of a life, liberty, or property interest, the person must be given notice, the opportunity to be heard, and a decision by a neutral decision maker. https://www.law.cornell.edu/wex

Punitive damages: Awarded in addition to actual damages in certain circumstances and considered punishment. Typically, punitive damages are awarded at the court's discretion when the defendant's behavior is found to be especially harmful.

Qualified immunity: A type of legal immunity that balances two important interests—the need to hold public officials accountable when they exercise power irresponsibly and the need to shield officials from harassment, distraction, and liability when they perform their duties reasonably.

Recidivism: Refers to a person's relapse into criminal behavior, often after the person receives sanctions or undergoes intervention for a previous crime.

Redacted: To cut out, white-out, or black-out parts of a document. In legal proceedings, this is generally justified for reasons of privilege.

Remand: To send back to the lower court.

Retribution: Punishment inflicted on someone as vengeance for a wrong or criminal act.

Ripeness: A claim is "ripe" when the facts of the case have matured into an existing substantial controversy warranting judicial intervention.

Standard of proof: Degree of proof required. In criminal cases, prosecutors must prove a defendant's guilt "beyond a reasonable doubt." The majority of civil lawsuits require proof "by a preponderance of the evidence" (50% plus), but in some the standard is higher and requires "clear and convincing" proof. https://www.uscourts.gov/glossary

Standing: The capacity of a party to bring suit in court.

Stare decisis: Latin for "to stand by things decided." The term is used in case opinions to reference the doctrine of precedent.

Subpoena: A command, issued under a court's authority, to a witness to appear and give testimony.

Subpoena duces tecum: A command to a witness to appear and produce documents.

Substantive due process: Substantive due process is the notion that due process not only protects certain legal procedures, but also protects certain rights unrelated to procedure. https://www.law.cornell.edu/wex

Summary judgment motion: A motion to request the court to rule that the other party has no case, because there are no facts at issue. The party making the motion is claiming that either the case should not go before a jury at all, or a jury could only rule in favor of the moving party.

Tribunal: Generally, a special court chosen by a government or governments to examine a particular problem

Waiver: A unilateral act of one person that results in the surrender of a legal right. The right relinquished can be constitutional, statutory, or contractual but must be voluntarily surrendered. If voluntarily surrendered, it is considered an express waiver.

Writ of certiorari: An order issued by the U.S. Supreme Court directing the lower court to transmit records for a case which it will hear on appeal.

Writ of habeas corpus: Latin for "that you have the body." In the U.S. system, federal courts can use the writ of habeas corpus to determine if a state's detention of a prisoner is valid. A writ of habeas corpus is used to bring a prisoner or other detainee (e.g., institutionalized mental patient) before the court to determine if the person's imprisonment or detention is lawful. A habeas petition proceeds as a civil action against the State agent (usually a warden) who holds the defendant in custody. It can also be used to examine any extradition processes used, the amount of bail, and the jurisdiction of the court. https://www.law.cornell.edu/wex/habeas_corpus

INDEX

Note: Page numbers followed by *t* denote tables.

For the benefit of digital users, indexed terms that span two pages (e.g., 52–53) may, on occasion, appear on only one of those pages.

CPSIA information can be obtained
at www.ICGtesting.com
Printed in the USA
BVHW051135090723
666696BV00002B/7